Child and Adolescent Counselling with Expressive Therapies

AF839577

This practical guide to Expressive Therapies tools – a multi-modal, emotion-focused application of creative arts therapies – explains how expressive, creative and collaborative counselling methods can be offered to young people who experience emotional, behavioural, cognitive or existential difficulties.

The authors share insights, principles and practical activities that they have developed, applied clinically and subsequently researched and taught for over 35 years. Chapters detail information on empowering young clients to learn mindful reflection and communicate their internal experiences using visual art, music, drama, movement, use of miniatures and language. An integrative theoretical framework is provided that offers wide activity choices, responding to client preferences. Expressive Therapies aims to foster a clients' capacity for resilience, hope and optimism. The appetite for more experiential, multi-modal creative arts-based approaches has evolved due to a rapidly growing evidence base for effectiveness, as well as for providing multi-cultural support. This book fulfils that demand with over 70 age-appropriate creative arts therapeutic activities and a contemporary evidence base. Its consideration of multiple intelligence theory enhances client engagement and counsellor–client alliance, and boosts both therapist and client confidence.

With its combination of principles and theory and practical activities, this is an indispensable guide for mental health professionals including counsellors, social workers, creative arts therapists and psychologists. Occupational therapists and similar professionals will also benefit, as will lecturers and students of creative arts therapy approaches.

Mark Pearson, PhD, has been conducting courses in Expressive Therapies for over 35 years, was a counsellor for young clients for 28 years and lectured in counselling at four Australian universities for 20 years. He holds a PhD, a Master's in Education – Behaviour Management – and a Diploma in Teaching.

Helen Wilson, PhD, has over 35 years' experience as a counsellor and clinical supervisor and lectured in counselling at three Australian universities for 20 years. She holds a PhD, a Master's in Counselling and a Bachelor's degree in Human Resource Management.

Child and Adolescent Counselling with Expressive Therapies

Creative Arts Activities to Inspire Wellbeing

Mark Pearson and Helen Wilson

Routledge
Taylor & Francis Group
LONDON AND NEW YORK

Designed cover image: Mark Pearson

First published 2026
by Routledge
4 Park Square, Milton Park, Abingdon, Oxon OX14 4RN

and by Routledge
605 Third Avenue, New York, NY 10158

Routledge is an imprint of the Taylor & Francis Group, an informa business

© 2026 Mark Pearson and Helen Wilson

The right of Mark Pearson and Helen Wilson to be identified as authors of this work has been asserted in accordance with sections 77 and 78 of the Copyright, Designs and Patents Act 1988.

All rights reserved. No part of this book may be reprinted or reproduced or utilised in any form or by any electronic, mechanical, or other means, now known or hereafter invented, including photocopying and recording, or in any information storage or retrieval system, without permission in writing from the publishers.

For Product Safety Concerns and Information please contact our EU representative GPSR@taylorandfrancis.com. Taylor & Francis Verlag GmbH, Kaufingerstraße 24, 80331 München, Germany.

Trademark notice: Product or corporate names may be trademarks or registered trademarks, and are used only for identification and explanation without intent to infringe.

British Library Cataloguing-in-Publication Data
A catalogue record for this book is available from the British Library

Library of Congress Cataloging-in-Publication Data
Names: Pearson, Mark, 1950- author | Wilson, Helen, 1951- author
Title: Child and adolescent counselling with expressive therapies : creative arts activities to inspire wellbeing / Mark Pearson and Helen Wilson.
Description: Abingdon, Oxon ; New York, NY : Routledge, 2026. | Includes
bibliographical references and index. |
Identifiers: LCCN 2026001240 (print) | LCCN 2026001241 (ebook) | ISBN
9781041138617 hbk | ISBN 9781041138600 pbk | ISBN 9781003671879 ebk
Subjects: LCSH: Art therapy for children | Art therapy for youth | Arts--Therapeutic use
Classification: LCC RJ505.A7 P425 2026 (print) | LCC RJ505.A7 (ebook)
LC record available at https://lccn.loc.gov/2026001240
LC ebook record available at https://lccn.loc.gov/2026001241

ISBN: 9781041138617 (hbk)
ISBN: 9781041138600 (pbk)
ISBN: 9781003671879 (ebk)

DOI: 10.4324/9781003671879

Typeset in Galliard
by Deanta Global Publishing Services, Chennai, India

HW – For Lennox, India, Asher and Oakley

MP – For Grace, Zahana, Elke and Gael

Contents

Other Books by Pearson and Wilson

Pearson, M. (1991). *From healing to awakening: An introduction to transpersonal therapy*. Inner Work Partnership.

Pearson, M. (1997). *The healing journey: A workbook for self-discovery*. Lothian.

Pearson, M. (2004). *Emotional healing and self-esteem: Inner-life skills of relaxation, visualization and meditation for children and adolescents*. Jessica Kingsley Publishers.

Pearson, M. (2026). *Mindfulness and relaxation activities for all ages. 60 fun and engaging, evidence-based visualisations, meditations and self-awareness games*. Routledge.

Pearson, M., & Nolan, P. (1991). *Emotional first-aid for children: Emotional release exercises and inner-life skills*. Butterfly Books.

Pearson, M., & Nolan, P. (2004). *Emotional release for children: Repairing the past, preparing the future*. Jessica Kingsley Publishers.

Pearson, M., & Wilson, H. (2001). *Sandplay and symbol work: Emotional healing and personal development with children, adolescents and adults*. ACER Press.

Pearson, M., & Wilson, H. (2009). *Using expressive arts to work with mind, body and emotions: Theory and practice*. Jessica Kingsley Publishers.

The authors' peer-reviewed and research papers at: https://expressivetherapies.au/publications.php.

Figures

Activity Index

Foreword

This book introduces counselling with children and adolescents from 6 to 18 years of age and offers extended therapeutic options using Expressive Therapies (ET) tools largely developed by the authors since 1988. Although a common misconception is that creative arts therapies and play-based approaches are designed for children only, ET can support psychological and emotional growth and recovery in clients of all ages. The book offers theoretical principles, some of the growing evidence base, as well as over 70 practical multimodal ET activity formats, that give step-by-step guidance for presenters. The book follows the ET focus on both "how to be" with a client and generously provides much "to do" with a client.

This book addresses the question of what expressive, creative and collaborative counselling methods we can offer young people who experience emotional, behavioural, cognitive or existential challenges. The potential for ET to enhance effectiveness in the therapeutic encounter is also addressed. A range of ET modalities are described in addition to structured therapeutic activities, linked to the evidence base, as well as the "way of being" required for effective application.

The therapeutic activities have largely been developed, applied clinically and subsequently researched and taught by the authors in Australia for over 35 years. The book explores how an integrative view of a range of theoretical frameworks can support offering multiple activity choices, responding to client preferences. A unique contribution, introduced in this book, is the way consideration of multiple intelligence theory can be used practically to enhance client confidence, engagement and alliance.

1 Foundations of a Multi-Modal Creative Arts Practice

Introduction

As our lived environments become increasingly complex, support for mental wellbeing in young people is a more urgent task. Worldwide 10–20% of children and adolescents experience mental disorders (World Health Organization, n.d.). The World Health Organization notes that without treatment these conditions will severely influence a child's development, educational attainments and potential to live a fulfilling and productive life.

Mental wellbeing is a multi-dimensional construct: Mental health concerns can be wide-ranging and have complex origins, related to – among other life experiences – family, social and cultural issues (Midgley, Hayes & Cooper, 2017). A growing number of adolescents experience elevated levels of struggle, stress and anxiety (Watson & Lemon, 2011). They may struggle to make sense of their emotional, physical, social and psychological development (Westergaard, 2013). Guiding a child or adolescent to broaden their understanding of themselves and the intersection between their outer and inner worlds can have a direct, positive impact on the quality of their emotional and social life.

While we feel great satisfaction when we see positive outcomes, we realise not all young people are ready and willing to engage in therapy, and some remain in environments that can act against this. Creating conditions and activities that call out this readiness and willingness is the first task for every counsellor. Professional counselling can reduce stress, build psychological resilience, empower problem-solving and mitigate the impact of adverse childhood experiences (Pattison & Harris, 2006). Research shows that the four most often used approaches to counselling young people – cognitive-behavioural, person-centred, psychodynamic and creative therapies – are all effective across the full range of counselling issues (Pattison & Harris, 2006). What the research does not illuminate is the number of young clients who may not be able to engage well in therapy that depends primarily on verbal communication.

Expressive Therapies (ET) is a form of activity-based creative arts counselling and psychotherapy that makes space for emotional and somatic transformation.

DOI: 10.4324/9781003671879-1

ET practitioners work in the present, while the structure of the activities supports processing the past if needed. ET provides creative-arts-based activities that support resolution of emotional difficulties, exploration of beliefs, deepening somatic awareness and regulating behaviour. ET has been developed as a multi-modal counselling support for children, adolescents and adults. As you read on, you will notice that we like to include the early evidence base, as well as recent research. Early research (while no longer fashionable) was part of our foundations, and we respect the early explorers in our field.

Each young person has a unique way of expressing concerns, or holding back from expression, or seeking approval and acceptance from others. In therapy, a young client explores walking between two seemingly opposite ways of being. On the one hand, they may stridently resist being told how to be or what to do, and may demonstrate a desire to be uninhibited in their expressive capacities. On the other hand, they want to know how to find acceptance and validation for who they are and how they want to be in the world. They want to be heard, but may not know where to start. The task of a counsellor is to accept and "hold" these dichotomies.

Experiencing freedom to share their distress, or hold back until they feel safe, is crucial in the development of the therapeutic relationship. A challenge for a counsellor is to provide steps and strategies for client reflection and communication, and to sit attentively as a client grapples with their distress and the search for a starting point. Clients may also, at times, need acceptance to seek distraction, to temporarily digress from challenges. Once a therapeutic alliance has formed, the experience of being "accompanied" in the counselling process begins to free up psychological resources. This allows exploration, relating and creativity through exploring what is meaningful to the client (Badenoch, 2017).

There may be a time in the early stages of counselling when a child or adolescent client tends to hang on to the edge of the pool, fearful to let go and float into deeper water. In the desire to help, a counsellor may get busy offering suggestions, may begin to talk of consequences, or intervene with well-known evidence-based ways to alleviate frustration or feelings of stuckness. In their heart, a counsellor may truly desire that the young client be able to find a "happier place". Caution is advised, however, not to rush to fix or reframe. Can a therapist sit with a client in the space of not knowing, and temporarily "not doing"?

Respectful and effective therapy with young people requires an open mind, a sense of playfulness and broad flexibility in both response options and therapeutic activities. In addition, the ability to create a safe psychological space for a client is core to the process. In other words, how we are, and even who we are, as counsellors becomes instrumental in effectively supporting a young client. There is growing evidence of the importance of a counsellor's way of being with a young client. For example, Knight et al. (2018) found that the young participants in their study most wanted from their school counsellors was genuine connection, being listened to, and being believed in. Similarly, Gibson et al. (2016) found that a priority for young adolescent clients was being able to keep control, and to have a relationship with their counsellor that was more like a friendship, to be listened to, and to feel they could talk freely.

Counselling for a young person, if based purely on the application of formulaic or manualised therapy models, may not meet the needs of the moment, nor bring engagement and the desired outcomes. Having something to "do", having a therapeutic activity, and someone to witness that doing, means the young person becomes an active participant in their own healing process.

While this book offers over 70 therapeutic activities, options for a large amount of "doing", the authors emphasise that "being with" a client and following their unfolding process, discerning their preferences for engagement, is essential to set the scene for positive outcomes.

What Is Expressive Therapies?

The ET approach described here includes a flexible and interactive range of activities to explore, process and resolve causes of emotional distress, which can shape the interior landscape and influence behaviour. ET includes use of somatic and emotional focus, visual art, music, metaphor, movement, therapeutic writing, drama, miniatures, relaxation, visualisation and mindfulness practice. Process-oriented, with an invitation to self-discovery through a person-centred relationship, ET aims to foster a client's capacity for resilience, hope and optimism.

Significantly, the way of being with clients, the willingness to be in the client's not knowing space, in addition to our understanding of, and expertise with the methods, contributes to forming and maintaining the therapeutic alliance. The evidence has been clear for some time that this alliance is a significant contributor to positive outcomes (Ardito & Rabellino, 2011). The positive relationship between alliance and outcomes was found to be consistent across the literature (Martin et al., 2000).

ET integrates the strengths of many approaches to form pluralistic, flexible, creative arts-based, experiential activities. Engagement with creative arts can bridge known and unknown issues and capacities, in addition to providing direct reconnection with a wider range of internal resources. Resilience emerges from a client's development of their Inner-Life Skills (see more on page 180). These skills are enhanced through engagement with ET, and include the development of emotional literacy, as well as ways to understand and manage their inner and outer worlds.

Activity-based ET sessions can bring resolution and integration through a reconnection between body, mind, feelings and behaviour. Sessions are intended to cooperate with a natural movement within the psyche towards healing and wholeness. This is a developmental process Jung named as individuation, Maslow identified as self-actualising and was considered by Rogers

(1967) as an underlying tendency towards self-development and functioning with autonomy. Challenges are likely to be faced when a client's own growth and development clash with family or cultural norms, challenges that are a normal part of development. In short, this means counsellors can support this natural process for young people, with confidential, flexible and multi-modal activities.

Therapeutic success has been attributed to clients' "active self-healing" tendencies, in addition to a therapist's role in freeing up a client's innate tendency to grow, develop and heal (Bohart, 2000; Bohart & Tallman, 1999; McVeigh, 2022). An aim of ET sessions is to activate an innate healing drive in the psyche, which, given the right conditions of safety, support and trust, can positively guide the therapeutic process. Primitive versions of this drive can be observed in the particular ways a client acts out or withdraws.

ET is a client-centred approach; that is, therapy progresses with respect for the client's speed and direction of the therapeutic process. Counsellors learn the dance between creating conditions or contexts for leading, focusing, directing clients and providing freedom, while being sensitive to follow a client's timing and preferences. These conditions support sustainable change in the client.

Safety

Therapy works best if a young person is able to feel physically and psychologically safe, within an encouraging and confidential therapeutic context. As within secure attachment, acceptance means a client is more willing to explore, experiment and discover. When entering a counselling process that provides an experience of acceptance, a judgement-free atmosphere, where the pressure of logic and outcomes can be temporarily suspended, clients can feel heard, their suffering seen and, to an increasing degree, they can allow themselves to be "found", to be known and knowable. They need to feel the therapist seeks to know who they are, has time to listen, is willing to explore their questions and concerns around anxiety, fear and identity. To feel safe, they need to experience a context of warmth and willingness to encounter who they are beyond the presenting problem.

Clients with limited communication skills, who engage with the range of creative activities of ET, can feel that what they have to say, and who they are, is communicated and experienced as having value, purpose and meaning. What is conveyed is that therapy is not merely a resolution of problems but acts as support for the creation of self-understanding and multiple ways for clients to tell their stories, and then move into creative and optimistic problem-solving.

Choice

Being able to have choice of discussion topics, how they relate to a counsellor, and which activities are preferred, all provide a sense of control and construct the encounter in a way that makes it easier to move forward. ET aims to provide activities that are a container for processing distress and making sense of the world. ET activities provide a regulating balance of freedom and structure, along with inbuilt scaffolding to enhance effective reflection and communication. The collaboration that brings freedom and choice within the therapeutic setting situates ET within a contemporary pluralistic practice.

Play

A capacity and willingness to create an atmosphere of play is essential for engagement. Play, or openness to spontaneity with ideas and methods, supports being able to choose from among a wide range of therapeutic activities. Clients thrive with permission to be spontaneous, or with time to reflect and rehearse what they feel able to share or disclose. And, as with adult therapy, accommodation of their preferences can lead to engagement and readiness to address concerns (Swift et al., 2013).

Which Way to Go? Where to Start? What Do Clients Need?

There are a broad range of therapeutic approaches to support young clients. Some were originally developed as stand alone techniques. The current focus, however, is a more integrated system that engages the client, one that allows recognition of what Cooper (2019) calls directionality. What directionality implies is a need for differing methods that achieve the changing therapeutic goals that emerge along a client's therapeutic journey. For example, the early stages of therapy benefit from active listening, middle stages might require – in order to help clients find their direction – self-awareness and self-discovery activities, whereas later stages may need problem-solving and formulation of revised strategies (Cooper, 2019). The challenge is to apply the most useful or relevant approach for each client, at each stage of their therapy. From a wide range of ET activities, a counsellor offers the most appropriate and relevant combination of expressive, somatic, cognitive, behavioural, emotional, or existential exploration. And these are offered within the distinct ET 5-Stage Model (see p. 36).

The hoped-for outcome for a young client is a deepening of self-awareness, increased capacity for self-reflection and greater freedom in productive self-expression, that can lead to enhanced self-regulation. The aim is to stimulate, amplify and contain a client's therapeutic process in an age-appropriate and supportive way (Kim et al., 2011). One of the elegant outcomes of using ET is that the client can "experience" themselves, their voice is given space and recognition, and they receive validating feedback, not just from a counsellor, but reflected back from their own creative expression. The process of self-discovery helps consolidate an emerging identity, along with self-management skills. Clients become the creator and interpreter of their response to any particular ET activity. This is one of the ways free creative expression, within therapy, can crystallise issues clients have some awareness of, as well as bringing to light memories, feelings, core beliefs that may linger out of sight. Explicit and implicit experiences can come together, revealing a fuller picture, leading to new options.

Contemporary counselling embraces potential for effectiveness from sources such as theoretical frameworks, a broad range of techniques and ways of interacting with a client that are most relevant to the moment. Strengths can be discovered in all approaches. There is, however, a challenge to intentionally integrate what is most effective for the client sitting before us and their needs in the moment. This may mean that even if we regard ourselves as expressive or creative arts therapists, there may be times when it is most appropriate to work with our client on problem-solving, or addressing unhelpful thinking patterns, talking or not talking, moving or being still, being spontaneous and creative, or planning, focusing on the moment, or dreaming up solutions that can then be closely examined.

Pluralism: An Integrative Foundation

For some readers new to ET, it may initially seem that we are swimming in a sea of theory and methods, with odd currents pushing this way and that. The theoretical framework that brings order to the options and possibilities ET offers comes from the work of Cooper and McLeod's (2011) pluralistic approach to counselling and psychotherapy. This is a logical extension of Rogers' person-centred therapy, and has been attracting a growing following, particularly in the UK and Europe. The focus is on the ethical necessity of responding to client diversity and preferences, and providing respect for clients' views on what may best help them (read more here: https://pluralisticpractice.com/).

Pluralism developed as an alternative to belief in a single approach to the psyche and refers to the notion that a number of valid responses or answers can be found to significant questions and "different things are likely to help different people at different points in time" (Cooper & McLeod, 2010, p. 3). Research has indicated that client retention and therapeutic outcomes are enhanced through responding to client preferences (Swift et al., 2013). This endorses the pluralistic practice of involving clients in discussions of preferred activities in the therapy room (Cooper & McLeod, 2012). ET practitioners would ideally be open to a collaborative investigation into the best fit for each therapeutic mode for each client. We will introduce Gardner's (2006) theory of multiple intelligences (MI) and its contribution to understanding client preferences (see pages 8–12). At the heart of the pluralistic approach, there is a collaborative style of working, joint decision-making, and problem-solving between counsellor and client, based on transparency of ideas, viewpoints and methods offered.

There is a vast array of approaches to counselling and psychotherapy. Twenty years ago, Norcross (2005) estimated that there were more than 400 types of therapy, all with differing practices, techniques, foundations and perspectives on responding to psychological distress. Duncan et al. (2004) provided an even higher estimate, suggesting there are up to 1,000 different treatment models and techniques. So, how do we decide how to best support clients? Research has shown that some therapists just apply what they know or like, without surveying what clients need or want (Poznanski & McLennan, 2004).

Historically, counselling and psychotherapy were structured around separate sets of ideas and models, each with their own manuals, teaching schools and professional associations (McLeod, 2013). It was found, however, that adhering to one particular school can lead to closing off to the clinical activities of other therapeutic approaches and the significance of the therapeutic alliance (e.g., Crawford et al., 2002; Gershefski et al., 1996). This may incline a therapist to privilege adherence to method over sensitivity to client preferences, needs and collaborations. Diversification can, however, foster growth and creativity in counselling and psychotherapy (Cooper & McLeod, 2010, 2011). Flexibility in therapist attitude, in approach and in activities offered, is ideal for responding to the varying moods, needs and goals of young clients.

Cooper and McLeod (2007, 2010, 2011) identified the necessity of responding to client diversity using an appropriate range of therapeutic methods, collaborating with clients and providing recommendations for engagement in a wide range of extra-therapeutic activities beyond the consulting room, "cultural resources" that have been found to have mental health benefits. The pluralistic rationale is an ethical one: To strive for a humanistic, respectful agenda in which clients are most valued (Cooper & McLeod, 2012). This dynamic relationship could be considered an evolution of a respectful humanistic viewpoint, found in several other approaches. For example, some strength-based approaches and dialectical behaviour therapy work to ensure collaboration.

Collaboration is one way to deal with the likely power imbalance within adult-to-child professional relationships, and has also been shown to be essential in forming an alliance with mandated clients (Bergner, 2019), as young clients most often are at first. Expressive therapists have a large "counselling menu", providing multiple options for therapeutic activities. Responding to client choice supports the client's experience of being respected.

Given the inevitable initial ambivalence that many young clients can present with, it is essential to be guided by clients' interests, abilities and enthusiasms. Likewise, helping young clients identify, articulate and work towards their immediate and wider life goals will be central. This may counteract their presumption that parents' or carers' goals could be those guiding a therapist. Initially, life goals may reflect broad desires, for example, "I want to feel good about myself". With a life goal as the foundation, we may gradually help a client identify some specific, explicit goals with tangible starting points. For some clients, testing out therapy may be a first goal, and this may include testing the counsellor, to see how patient and trustworthy they are. Once rapport and trust goals are resolved, the next level of specific goals can be shared, for example: *I want to be less worried about school work. I want to stop my angry outbursts,* etc.

This book provides scripts for a wide variety of practical activities that can expand a counsellor's available methods. ET provides many catalysts for client reflection and conversation, ways to concretise problem-solving, multiple ways of providing new experiences of self, or identifying strengths and – cherished in a pluralistic approach – encouragement for the client to integrate extra-therapeutic resources for mental health, through "homework" suggestions.

Multiple Intelligence Theory

As research findings are inevitably generalised to a large degree, we are fond of pointing out to counselling students that, despite the abundance of research, "there is no research which tells you what will work best for the person sitting in front of you". Effective counsellors are required to become everyday researchers, at the micro level, aiming to discover afresh doorways into the psyche of today's client.

An approach to counselling that incorporates multiple intelligence (MI) theory and practice (O'Brien & Burnett, 2000; Pearson, 2011; Pearson et al., 2015) suggests that an assessment of client "strengths" or preferred intelligences can provide a platform for collaboration, a starting point for therapy. This, in turn, assists the selection of client-favoured therapy methods and is specifically useful in the early stages of alliance formation. Multiple intelligence (MI) theory (Gardner, 1983, 2006) and its application to counselling have been a key interest for us (e.g., Pearson, 2011; Pearson et al., 2015). MI can provide a way to discern among the array of creative arts approaches what might make the best sense to our client.

This MI contribution towards pluralistic practice has been referred to by McLeod (2018) as providing "epistemic fluidity" (p. 27), or support for identifying client "ways of knowing". He described counsellors and clients as having five contrasting sources of knowledge (theoretical, practical, cultural, personal and scientific). MI can use all these. McLeod (2018) suggested that "the most effective problem-solving occurs when dialogue takes place between different ways of knowing" (p. 26).

Harvard researcher, Professor Howard Gardner, first described his original seven-intelligence MI theory in 1983. MI theory became instrumental in school curriculum planning and was widely adopted in the field of education, with outcomes of increased student awareness about the learning process, stimulation of the learning process, increased student motivation, reduction in behavioural disruptions, increases in self-esteem and improvements in teacher–pupil relationships (Hopper & Hurry, 2000). Gardner deliberately used the term "intelligence" to identify what could also be referred to as "faculties" or "gifts", and has stated that he is also willing to call them "talents" or "abilities" (Visser et al., 2006).

The use of an MI framework as a support for, and within, counselling and psychotherapy with young people has been suggested by Bowles (2013), Keates and Pearson (2024), O'Brien and Burnett (2000), Pearson and O'Brien (2012), Pearson (2011) and Booth and O'Brien (2008). A study by O'Brien and Burnett (2000) examined the effectiveness of implementing an MI approach to school counselling with primary students. A single quantitative study (Bowles, 2013) investigated adult therapy clients' perceptions of their MI talents as they began therapy, although MI was not used in treatment. Further to this, Chan (2001) suggested that applying MI in the psychological counselling of students could achieve an integration of talent development and personal growth. Chan found that MI can be used through integration of creative arts processes into counselling.

MI theory has significant implications for supporting quality counselling, approaches that can respond to and possibly expand each client's individual intelligence profile. Additionally, MI theory provides a framework for integrating many styles of counselling into an individually meaningful meta-approach.

Contemporary MI theory delineates eight distinct – possibly nine – intelligences, each one representing a different way that people can reflect, communicate and learn. The intelligences can be summarised as verbal linguistic (strong ability to use words), logical mathematical (ability with deductive reasoning), visual spatial (ability to use images and graphic designs), musical rhythmic (ability to express through music and rhythm), bodily kinaesthetic (ability with movement and use of the body), intrapersonal (awareness of internal moods and thoughts – also termed by others emotional intelligence [e.g., Mayer & Salovey, 1995]), interpersonal (ability to learn and express through relating to others) and naturalistic environmental (affinity with nature and living things) (Nolen, 2003). Additionally, Gardner (1999) proposed a possible existential intelligence (being concerned with reflection on transcendental concerns, such as the significance of life or the meaning of death).

Counsellors are traditionally trained to focus on the application of verbal/linguistic intelligence (questioning, communicating issues and telling the story) and logical/mathematical intelligence (through engaging cognitive problem-solving and reviewing consequences of behaviour). Using an MI approach to counselling may be more effective and lead to more positive outcomes for clients whose preferred intelligences during counselling differ from the traditional verbal linguistic and logical mathematical intelligence (Booth & O'Brien, 2008). Many styles of therapy have come to specialise in one or two of the intelligences. If utilising more of the intelligences in education results in quality education, could initiating access to a broader range of intelligences in counselling result in increased quality of service and therapeutic effectiveness?

MI and Counselling Approaches

MI theory sheds some light on possible reasons for the evolution of such a wide range of therapeutic orientations and modalities. Are new approaches developed from an understanding of client's intelligence preferences, or could counsellors' and researchers' own intelligence preferences guide this process? Let's look at the way the intelligences are used in the fields of counselling and psychotherapy.

Verbal/linguistic Intelligence: This has been at the heart of Western psychotherapy. Freud adopted the term "the talking cure" to describe psychoanalysis (Freud, 1910/1995). This intelligence is utilised in verbal therapy, therapeutic writing and bibliotherapy. Clients who think and learn through written and spoken words, and have the ability to memorise facts, fill in workbooks, respond to written tasks and enjoy reading, may prefer or respond more positively to this style of activity.

Musical/Rhythmic Intelligence: This would be utilised when spontaneous music-making, rhythm-making, or recorded music is used as part of therapy. It can be connected with the kinaesthetic intelligence through dance to rhythms, and to the verbal/linguistic intelligence through the rhythms of poetry used in, or as, therapy. The musical/rhythmic intelligence is ideal for clients who can recognise tonal patterns and environmental sounds, and who learn through rhyme, rhythm and repetition.

Logical/Mathematical Intelligence: This is widely used in cognitive behavioural therapy and programmes that use applied behaviour analysis. Approaches that use the logical/mathematical intelligence may be most helpful for clients who emphasise the cognitive aspect of their life, who can think deductively, deal with consequences, numbers and recognise patterns.

Interpersonal Intelligence: This is the ability to understand others and work effectively with them. It underlies the development of the therapeutic alliance, given that almost all approaches to counselling utilise interpersonal connections. The well-researched person-centred approach (Rogers, 1951) focuses on creating a safe, respectful and positive interpersonal connection. In the person-centred style of counselling, the activation of interpersonal intelligence is central. Interpersonal intelligence is in action in clients who communicate and learn and operate best one-to-one, as well as through group relationships.

Visual/Spatial Intelligence: At the core of art therapy and the use of drawing, mind maps, collage, sandplay therapy and symbol work is the visual/spatial intelligence. While a wide range of clients are able to express and communicate via arts-based modalities, they are particularly useful for clients who can think with and visualise images and pictures. In addition, a client who utilises this intelligence demonstrates an ability to create graphic designs and communicate with diagrams, images and symbols.

Bodily/Kinaesthetic Intelligence: This refers to an ability with sensory awareness and movement, as utilised in somatically focused therapies, dance/movement therapy, bioenergetics and relaxation. Clients for whom these modalities are attractive can learn through physical movement and body wisdom, and may have a sense of knowing through body memory. Access to sensory clues to internal processes is another characteristic of the bodily/kinaesthetic intelligence.

Naturalist Intelligence: This is developed, encouraged and utilised in approaches that employ connection to nature, ecopsychology, horticultural therapy, as well as through therapeutic use of relating with pets, for example, equine assisted therapy. This intelligence involves an ability to recognise categories in nature, and sensitivity to natural phenomena.

Intrapersonal Intelligence: This is highly utilised in a psychodynamically oriented approach to counselling, in ET, in emotion-focused therapy and in the use of visualisation and meditation. Skills in this area are integral components of mental wellbeing (Kaufhold & Johnson, 2005), in addition to being central in effective engagement in learning (Shepard et al., 1999). A client with a preference for the intrapersonal might enjoy and learn through self-reflection, participate in metacognition and like working alone.

Existential (The Proposed Ninth Intelligence): This has been more popularly labelled as a "spiritual intelligence", although Gardner (2000) argued against the use of this term. The existential intelligence would include the ability to contemplate metaphysical concepts and deal with "questions beyond sensory data" (Moran et al., 2006, p. 24). Use of this proposed intelligence and associated activities (such as spiritual reflection, meditation, prayer) is central to transpersonal psychotherapy, existential therapy and therapies that utilise spiritual or religious techniques.

One of the tasks for a counsellor working within a pluralistic framework is to discover and initially work with techniques that utilise the intelligences with which a client is most naturally adept. Beginning with the natural or preferred intelligence and related communication style, the goal, depending on client tolerance, would be to eventually offer activities that stimulate intelligences and skills that have been used less often. This varying of intelligences used builds a client's sense of competence and allows them to communicate, and more easily work through issues in a way that is experienced as non-threatening and non-oppositional (O'Brien & Burnett, 2000).

O'Brien and Burnett (2000) found that the most often used intelligence by student clients was the interpersonal, followed by the bodily/kinaesthetic, then the visual/spatial. According to their findings, the logical/mathematical intelligence was the least preferred with young behaviour-challenged clients.

We have found that ET activities can have a positive and profound impact in supporting young clients when we consider their natural intelligences and abilities. ET invites reflection on, and safe expression of, emotion in ways that may not occur within traditional verbal exchanges. ET is one approach that provides a counsellor and client with opportunities to respond creatively to a variety of abilities, traits and intelligences.

The Intrapersonal or Emotional Intelligence

Gardner (2006) described the intrapersonal intelligence as concerning access to one's feeling life, the capacity to represent feelings and the ability to draw on them as a means of understanding, and as a guide for behaviour. This reminds us of Greenberg's (2002) concept of supporting clients to harness emotions as guides. The intrapersonal intelligence can act as a hub and has an integrative role in relation to the other intelligences (O'Brien & Burnett, 2000b). In the field of counselling, particularly in psychodynamically oriented and emotion-focused approaches, it may be the activation and use of the intrapersonal intelligence that can account for much of the insight and growth for clients.

Linking emotional intelligence and therapy, Mayer and Salovey (1995) identified that defences against emotion (such as denial, projection and intellectualisation) may impede judgement because they reduce both "pain" and the information about the world that accompanies it. Increased defensiveness (and closing off of information) may lead to reduced sensitivity to others, less social understanding and even poorer health (Mayer & Salovey, 1995). Engaging clients in the use of intrapersonal intelligence is sometimes met with initial resistance. However, using MI strategies lowered resistance and "diminished the impact of the ego defences", and the use of visual/spatial intelligence often led to some discussion of intrapersonal problems (O'Brien & Burnett, 2000, p. 153).

Assessing Natural or Preferred Intelligences

To inform themselves about their own and their clients' natural or preferred intelligences, and the possible intelligence assumptions underlying their professional work, counsellors have access to a number of MI preference tests (e.g., Chislett & Chapman, 2005; McKenzie, 1999; Shearer, 1996). Another widely used scale, designed for school students, that utilises images as well as text, is the Teele Inventory for Multiple Intelligences (TIMI) (Teele, 1992). This scale provides an opportunity to gauge young people's perceptions of their own intelligence preferences.

For work with young clients Connell's (2005) MI questionnaire (pdf free on the internet), developed for the classroom, can provide young clients and their counsellors with a guide to possible preferences. Of course, direct observation of the client and developing conversations, during initial sessions, that explore cognitive abilities and general interests may provide clear clues as to client intelligence preferences. However, the assessment scales may both support these conversations and provide speedy feedback, and become catalysts for generating collaboration. Offering appropriate MI counselling activities allows counsellors to respond in an informed, flexible and practical way to client needs, abilities and interests.

What Does ET Practice Look Like?

Enhancing therapeutic effectiveness requires the expressive therapist to be skilled at both doing and being. Therapy provides a combination of action supported by a quiet, concentrated presence on the part of the counsellor. A brief overview of the processes of ET provides a sense of the experience and structure of a session. Our Five-Stage Session Model is addressed in more detail in Chapter 2, detailed on page 36.

As is the case for all therapeutic models, the development of initial rapport within a hoped-for therapeutic alliance, experienced by a client as warm, caring, flexible, non-judgemental and workable, is required in order to build trust. Young clients are almost always mandated clients, so often the initial challenge is to support them to move from mandated attendance to enthusiastic participation. ET invites contact and collaboration between the client and their chosen activity. This is then followed by the provision of options within a broad range of expressive activities to help a client clarify and externalise their internal experience, to identify and clarify their thoughts, feelings, somatic and energetic states and behavioural drives.

Therapist Skills in Being Present

Therapist presence has been recognised as a major contributor to rapport-building and positive therapy outcomes (e.g., Dunn et al., 2013; Geller & Greenberg, 2012). Many of our young clients feel that no one listens, that they do not matter, and it seems like a revelation when they realise we are paying attention, interested, focused and curious to learn who they are, in a judgement-free environment. Our primary rule in starting out with a new client is to meet the client "where they are". We need to let go of self-criticism if clients are unsure of their readiness to engage or self-protect; if they seem to open, then close, focus then quickly distract themselves. We need to be prepared, to plan for sessions, and at the same time remain flexible to follow the client's unfolding process, their interests, with patience.

Principles and Practices of ET

Training: For counsellors adopting ET, involvement in experiential and transformational learning and personal development opportunities, incorporating a range of creative arts modalities, is crucial. This background informs selecting and using the activities safely and creating safety and permission for clients' experience within sessions. Having a training experience that values the evidence base and challenges and expands conceptual frameworks is essential. We don't offer a client an activity we have not explored personally. We don't invite them to go where we have not been.

Therapeutic Flexibility: ET tailors therapeutic activities to meet the client's needs, abilities and preferences. In collaboration with the client, ET provides activities which respect their abilities and intelligence strengths. An important counsellor skill is the flexibility to flow, or pivot, between modalities in order to meet the client's needs. This supports finding the most available "doorway" into their inner life. One day the doorway may be art, one day it may be emotion, and in the next session there could be a focus on behaviour strategies. ET also supports the client's awareness to move between the known and the unknown, the inner and outer, the explicit and implicit.

Acting-Out vs Active Therapy: Boundaries between expressive activities in the therapy room that may involve role-play and at times some degree of venting, and acting-out behaviours in daily life, need to be clear and repeated. If clients can process reactive emotions that drive behaviour in privacy, in a way that no one is offended, the tendency or need to act out in daily life is decreased. There is then the opportunity to access underlying vulnerable, primary feelings (more on this in Chapter 7). Feeling safe to experience vulnerability can have a dramatic effect in reducing impulses towards acting-out.

Hold Interpretations Lightly: Sharing your interpretations of an individual's inner world of thoughts, beliefs, metaphors and imagery represented symbolically can decrease their self-discovery, self-efficacy and positive outcomes. It is normal practice for a counsellor not to assume any specific or standardised meanings are attached to any symbols, metaphors, drawings, use of colours, dreams or fantasy images a client might share. There are times when a client's symbolic thinking or symbolic artefacts can bring swift insight, and there are many times when explicit meanings remain a mystery. The counsellor's role is not to solve the mystery or resolve the tension of not knowing, but to support curiosity.

Client Self-Awareness: Cognitive, emotional and somatic awareness is enhanced by encouraging clients to turn their focus internally and take some deep breaths. Many ET activities encourage clients to open breath and deepen self-awareness. Through developing enhanced awareness clients can better gauge internal forces that could lead to unwanted behaviours. Through developing enhanced awareness clients can come to better understand emotions and somatic signals and are more likely to have choice in their responses to the world. Development of emotional and somatic awareness increases overall emotional intelligence, and this can become a valuable life-long asset.

Mechanisms of Emotion-Focused Recovery: Present ET to clients as a journey towards growth, emotional maturity, a positive sense of self, rather than just a problem-solving exercise. The natural state of healthy emotions is expression, flow and transformation. Acknowledging and experiencing emotions and, when appropriate, expressing them, enhances mental health and reduces reactive behaviour. Since emotional integration is also a somatic event, help clients become more aware of their internal sensory experiences.

The Inner Healer

Through his long career studying the human psyche, Jung identified a natural in-built, logical drive towards mental health and wholeness. This mechanism is referred to by some as the "inner healer", (e.g., a term used by Grof and Grof [2010] to denote an intrinsic internal guiding mechanism that seeks psychological healing and wholeness). "Active self-healing" tendencies have been identified by several writers (e.g., Bohart, 2000; Bohart & Tallman, 1999; McVeigh, 2022). While there are many websites offering ways to awaken and connect with your inner healer, and several medical-related articles by nurse researchers (e.g., Dossey, 1991; Koithan, 2009), the concept has barely entered mainstream counselling.

Core to our flexibility in "doing" and "being" with a client is developing our capacity to trust in our client's innate healing mechanism. From the principles of Maslow's self-actualising clinical observations (1970), Roger's Person-Centred Therapy (Di Malta et al, 2024), as well as from the field of Transpersonal Psychotherapy (Rodrigues & Friedman, 2013), we adopt the notion of each person embodying an inbuilt self-actualising, homeostatic healing tendency. Alongi and Wade (2024) describe this broadly as the client being in the driver's seat. The simple process of collaboration with a client's internal healing tendency requires a therapist to be open, interested in the logic of how and when a client moves towards resolution of conflicts, and readiness to support any connection with, and expression of, emotion. Core to our flexible responding is being able to offer choice in action or stillness, activities or reflection time, and finding the client's preferred natural strengths in terms of multiple intelligences (see more on page 11).

We have debated ways to express the concept of an inner healer in less "alternative" sounding ways, but actually we find this term really fits, and most importantly it makes sense to clients. The concept supports clients to trust, or take seriously, their interoception, and attend to guidance from feelings and somatic signals. Stepping out of the way of ego-driven, conditioned, conscious decisions can in some cases allow self-discovery and self-guidance, that not only builds resilience but leads to more successful therapeutic integration.

This mechanism of the psyche selectively attunes the attentive client not only with what needs to be remembered, felt, released or integrated, but also with the timing that is individually appropriate. Effectiveness in the therapeutic process can be reduced if the counsellor has a pre-set agenda, for example, if following an overly manualised approach. Highly manualised interventions were viewed as negatively impacting therapeutic relationships, and over time having a detrimental effect on the therapist, in a study by Talens (2024). Gaining trust in an internal healing direction through experiential learning will allow a therapist to trust a client's preferences, choices, timing, direction and level of engagement.

What supports this intrinsic self-healing direction? Beginning to return to emotional and somatic flow increases discernment that allows self-direction.

The inner healer can become more active, or more obvious, when a client feels safe and accepted, when they gain trust in the counsellor, as well as in their own perceptions. Tapping into this drive is closely related to awakening an interest in self-discovery. For many clients, self-discovery and self-understanding have been buried under disappointment, distress and external approval seeking. Self-discovery forms the basis for the client to cooperate more willingly with their drive towards healing and wholeness, and counsellors' attention and acceptance can support this interest to re-surface.

A Growing Evidence Base

There are many types of evidence. Quite rightly, agencies and funding bodies are more often requiring that counsellors engage in evidence-based practice. In academic circles there is a notion that only randomised controlled trials (RCTs) count as evidence, and so approaches to counselling that are backed by these studies are assumed to be superior. However, the American Psychological Association states "Evidence-based practice is the integration of the best available research with clinical expertise in the context of patient characteristics, culture and preferences" (Evidence-Based Practice in Psychology (apa.org)). Obviously, the application of an approach without clinical expertise is meaningless, and consideration of individual client needs and preferences is essential. We often remark to counselling students that there is no accurate evidence for what is best for the person sitting in front of you, since research is largely general. Finding what works for your client today is a counsellor's ongoing research project, their life-long quest.

As well as formal research projects, the clinical observations and learnings from experienced therapists can inform our work. Some of the evidence we base our work on emerged from many years of clinical work, clinical supervision and the sharing of observations and discoveries through conferences and books and papers. Some of the research areas that can provide guidance and affirmation of practice that we will briefly mention include interpersonal neuroscience, trauma recovery, as well as depression and anxiety outcome studies. Within the creative arts therapies research, there are findings from individual and multiple case studies at one end of the spectrum, and RCTs and meta-analyses of past studies at the other end. Research on pluralistic practice is rapidly emerging, and this field is most relevant to ET.

An Informal Exploration of the Evidence – Expressive Therapies (2014–2025)

While we have woven reference to the ET evidence base throughout this book, here is an informal browse through the multi-modal ET literature from the last eleven years. There is also a vast array of evidence in relation to ET used with adult clients; however, we have not reviewed this here. While many of the individual creative arts therapy modalities have significant evidence bases established, here we focus on some of the emerging evidence for the integrated, multi-modal ET approach. One aspect that stands out from the literature is that ET is a global phenomenon.

Understandably, there are limited articles that explore outcomes from an integrated approach, in which an experienced therapist, supporting a real client, weaves together therapeutic arts activities in a flexible way that suits the specific needs of that client in the moment. In some literature, following a manual for application of a modality is considered a research strength. However, in practice, following a therapy manual, as opposed to spontaneously responding to client interests and needs, could turn out to be poor therapy.

We can find literature that emerges from all around the globe: Australia, China, Finland, Malaysia, Taiwan, South Africa, South Korea, Thailand, Turkey, India, Venezuela, the Czech Republic, the UK and the USA. This confirms that ET is inherently a multicultural approach. Additionally, France (2020) demonstrates the healing power of the creative arts in therapy from a Canadian Indigenous perspective, and Graham (2013) recommends ET as a preferred trauma treatment option for Australian Aboriginal clients.

Mark's early article (Pearson, 2003), pointed to the overall effectiveness of ET used in Australian schools, with significant increases observed in positive emotional and behavioural outcomes and in motivation to attend counselling. Twenty guidance officers and counsellors from Australian schools, who had completed training in ET and had been integrating it into their professional work for between six months and five years, responded to a detailed qualitative questionnaire. Improvements, after the implementation of ET, were also apparent in the counsellor and client relationship. Two other earlier studies were based on our ET style: Booth and O'Brien (2008), and O'Brien and Burnett (2000), which both explored positive outcomes from using the multiple intelligences framework for applying ET with students. In reviewing approaches to support young people with anxiety (Keates & Pearson, 2024) a multiple intelligence and ET approach has been recommended.

We have recently described ways ET can support the development of rapport in counselling with young clients (Pearson & Wilson, 2024). In practice, effective relating requires activities that support the young client to gather their thoughts, identify their feelings and feel safe enough to discuss their behaviour. Within the last ten years we have found only one other study that specifically included our Australian style of ET used with young clients: This is Southwell's (2016) report on yourtown's ET intervention with 41 pre-school aged children impacted by developmental trauma and attachment problems. She describes an impressively flexible intervention that combines our style of ET (Pearson & Wilson, 2009), with child-centred play therapy, Perry's neurosequential model of therapeutics, Kalff's sandplay therapy and filial therapy.

Southwell reports: "Analysis of pre/post assessments of participants' social, emotional and behavioural functioning using the *Child Behaviour Checklist* revealed significant improvements from intake to exit in children's internalising, externalising and total problems. There were also marked decreases in the proportion of children with symptoms in the clinical or borderline clinical ranges. Thematic analyses of parent/carer surveys and therapists' end-of-therapy reports similarly indicate widespread improvements in social, emotional and behavioural functioning as well as improvements in children's self-confidence and self-esteem, and in the quality of the parent-child attachment relationship" (Southwell, 2016, p. 121).

The aim of a study by Çalık and Çelik (2019) was to investigate the effects of counselling programmes based on expressive activities with semi-structured groups on the self-concealment levels of adolescents. The results revealed that the "psychological counselling programme based on expressive activities with semi-structured groups" (p. 465) was significantly effective in alleviating self-concealment levels, and this effect was also maintained in follow-up evaluations four months later.

In the proceedings from a conference in the Czech Republic (Polínek & Telekyová, 2025) there is a description of how ET could be integrated into education. The paper argues for the systematic inclusion of expressive therapeutic and psychotherapeutic elements in school education, "not only in the field of cognitive learning development (e.g. mathematics, science), but especially in the field of mental health education, prevention of mental health problems and development of key social competences". The paper presents research demonstrating the positive impact of expressive approaches on the saturation of basic psychological needs and presents the results of a project that monitored the effectiveness of expressive-therapeutic interventions in the development of social behaviour and soft skills in second grade primary school pupils.

A literature review from India on ET (blending dance and movement, art therapy and music therapy) for survivors of child sexual abuse was conducted by Lavania and Ballal (2025). The literature indicated that ET offers a safe space for recovery that encourages hope, self-determination and healthy relationships. These approaches encourage cognitive processing, emotional expression and physical connectedness.

A six-session multi-modal expressive arts program (Siu & Chan, 2020), was implemented for 14 secondary school students who met criteria as underachievers. Quantitative data from teachers and students indicated an increase in behavioural and emotional engagement at the end of the programme. The indifference within participants on the issue of "underachieving" was brought to their awareness through the programme and led to more self-reflection.

A number of researchers have pointed to the ways ET can support overall resilience. A review by Kalaf and Plante (2020) suggests that ET can enhance young refugees' resilience. They describe how ET can develop "pathways to resilience" through incorporating creative play, storytelling, meaning-making, healing of trauma, belongingness, hope and community engagement. Pearson and de Bruin (2019) advocate a pluralistic approach to practice, incorporating multiple therapy orientations and self-discovery ET methods, that counsellors may call on to enhance client resilience, along ten targeted pathways.

Asthma is the most common chronic disease of childhood (Ozceker et al., 2023), and its management largely depends on compliance with therapy. The aim of a study by Ozceker et al. (2023) was to investigate the effects of an 8-week expressive art therapy programme on asthma control and quality of life of asthmatic children. Pulmonary function tests, asthma control tests and an asthma quality-of-life scale for children were performed before and after the programme. There were statistically significant increases in pulmonary function tests and improvement in the items of quality of life in the young patients after the programme.

A meta-analytical study by Cambra (2019) investigated the effectiveness of expressive therapeutic modalities, including play, art, music, sandplay, theatre and writing therapies, in helping children and adolescents cope with refugee trauma. Findings indicate that expressive therapeutic modalities are among the beneficial modalities to integrate with other trauma-informed approaches. The overall combined effect on all pre-post outcomes was medium. Stress yielded a high effect size. Wellbeing, internalising behaviours and externalising behaviours all yielded medium effect sizes.

Siegel et al. (2016) reported on a novel form of ET where children created and used "healing sock creatures", developed in a paediatric unit in the USA. The activity received enthusiastic support from hospital staff and family members as they noted that the children were calmer following therapy, as well as throughout their hospital stay. This pilot study assessed observer impressions of, and measured, changes in the children's mood. The results showed improvements in mood for children following therapy sessions, compared to children in a wait-list control group.

A study by Zakaria (2015) investigated patterns of catharsis when adolescent girls involved in delinquency used expressive arts in group counselling. Data was drawn from in-depth interviews, observations and analysis of participant artefacts. Participants identified that the use of creativity and art enabled them to reduce stress, stabilise emotions and provide release from the emotional disturbances that have been a part of their life.

A hospital study explored expressive therapists' experiences working in a paediatric unit during the COVID-19 lockdown (Lahue et al., 2023). They encountered advantages when using telehealth, such as increased engagement and increased space for processing, as well as challenges. A key finding from the study was noting the value of ET in facilitating emotional expression and the insight individuals gain through creative reflection.

References

Alongi, P., & Wade, J., (2024). Clients in the driver's seat, not asleep at the wheel: A qualitative study of the client role in transpersonal psychotherapy. *International Journal of Transpersonal Studies*. Advance Publication Archive.

Ardito, R. B., & Rabellino, D. (2011). Therapeutic alliance and outcome of psychotherapy: historical excursus, measurements, and prospects for research. *Frontiers in Psychology, 2*, 270.

Badenoch, B. (2017). *The heart of trauma: Healing the embodied in the context of relationships (Norton Series on Interpersonal Neurobiology)*. WW Norton & Company.

Bergner, R. M. (2019). Ideas for enabling involuntary clients to engage voluntarily in therapy. *Journal of Systemic Therapies, 38*(2), 20–34.

Bohart, A. C. (2000). The client is the most important common factor: Clients' self-healing capacities and psychotherapy. *Journal of Psychotherapy Integration, 10*, 127–149.

Bohart, A. C., & Tallman, K. (1999). *How clients make therapy work: The process of active self-healing*. American Psychological Association.

Booth, R., & O'Brien, P. (2008). An holistic approach for counsellors: Embracing multiple intelligences. *International Journal for the Advancement of Counselling, 3*(2), 79–92.

Bowles, T. (2013). Enhancing strength-based therapy by focusing on client's talents and concepts of learning. *Electronic Journal of Applied Psychology, 9*(1), 19–30.

Çalık, M., & Çelik, E. (2019). The effect of counselling programmes involving expressive activities with semi-structured groups on self-concealment levels of adolescents. *Counselling and Psychotherapy Research, 19*(4), 465–473.

Cambra, B. K. (2019). *The effect of expressive therapies on refugee children and adolescents: Meta-analytic findings* (Doctoral dissertation). Liberty University.

Chan, D. W. (2001). Reframing student counseling from the multiple-intelligence perspective: Integrating talent development and personal growth. *Asian Journal of Counselling, 8*(1), 69–85.

Chislett, V., & Chapman, A. (2005). Multiple intelligences test – Based on Howard Gardner's MI model. www.businessballs.com

Connell, J. D. (2005). *Brain-based strategies to reach every learner*. Scholastic Teaching Resources

Cooper, M. (2019). *Integrating counselling and psychotherapy. Directionality, synergy, and social change*. Sage.

Cooper, M., & McLeod, J. (2007). A pluralistic framework for counselling and psychotherapy: Implications for research. *Counselling and Psychotherapy Research, 7*(3), 135–143.

Cooper, M., & McLeod, J. (2010). *Pluralistic counselling and psychotherapy*. Sage Publications.

Cooper, M., & McLeod, J. (2011). Person-centered therapy: A pluralistic perspective. *Person-Centered & Experiential Psychotherapies, 10*(3), 210–223.

Cooper, M., & McLeod, J. (2012). From either/or to both/and: Developing a pluralistic approach to counselling and psychotherapy. *European Journal of Psychotherapy & Counselling, 14*(1), 5–17.

Crawford, M. J., Rutter, D., Manley, C., Weaver, T., Bhui, K., Fulop, N., & Tyrer, P. (2002). Systematic review of involving patients in the planning and development of health care. *British Medical Journal, 325*(7375), 1263–1267.

Di Malta, G., Cooper, M., O'Hara, M., Stephen, S., & Gololob, Y. (2024). *The handbook of person-centred psychotherapy and counselling*. Bloomsbury Publishing.

Dossey, B. (1991). Awakening the inner healer. *The American Journal of Nursing*, *91*(8), 31–34.
Duncan, B. L., Hubble, M. A., & Miller, S. D. (2004). Beyond integration: The triumph of outcome over process in clinical practice. *Psychotherapy in Australia*, *10*(2), 32–80.
Dunn, R., Callahan, J. L., Swift, J. K., & Ivanovic, M. (2013). Effects of pre-session centering for therapists on session presence and effectiveness. *Psychotherapy Research*, *23*(1), 78–85.
France, H. (2020). Creative arts and the indigenous healing circle within an indigenous context. *Canadian Journal of Counselling & Psychotherapy*, *54*(3), 413–429.
Freud, S. (1910/1995). *Five lectures on psychoanalysis*. Penguin
Gardner, H. (1983). *Frames of mind: The theory of multiple intelligences*. Basic Books.
Gardner, H. (1999). *Intelligence reframed: Multiple intelligences for the 21st century*. Basic Books.
Gardner, H. (2000). *Intelligence reframed: Multiple intelligences for the 21st century*. Hachette UK.
Gardner, H. (2006). *Multiple intelligences. New horizons*. Basic Books.
Geller, S. M., & Greenberg, L. S. (2012). *Therapeutic presence: A mindful approach to effective therapy*. American Psychological Association.
Gershefski, J. J., Arnkoff, D., Glass, C., & Elkin, I. (1996). Clients' perceptions of treatment for depression: I. Helpful aspects. *Psychotherapy Research*, *6*, 233–247.
Gibson, K., Cartwright, C., Kerrisk, K., Campbell, J., & Seymour, F. (2016). What young people want: A qualitative study of adolescents' priorities for engagement across psychological services. *Journal of Child and Family Studies*, *25*, 1057–1065.
Graham, J. S. (2013). Expressive therapy as a treatment preference for Aboriginal trauma. *Pimatisiwin: A Journal of Aboriginal and Indigenous Community Health*, *11*(3), 501–512.
Greenberg, L. S. (2002). *Emotion-focussed therapy: Coaching clients to work through their feelings*. American Psychological Association.
Grof, S. (1998). The cosmic game: Explorations of the frontiers of human consciousness. Suny Press.
Grof, S., & Grof, C. (2010). *Holotropic Breathwork. A new approach to self-exploration and therapy*. State University of New York.
Hopper, B., & Hurry, P. (2000). Learning the MI way: The effects on students' learning of using the theory of multiple intelligences. *Pastoral Care in Education*, *18*(4), 26–32.
Kalaf, L., & Plante, P. (2020). Restoring lost resources for young refugees: An integrative review of the resilience-building potential of expressive therapies. *Canadian Journal of Art Therapy*, *33*(1), 5–16.
Kaufhold, J. A., & Johnson, L. R. (2005). The analysis of the emotional intelligence skills and potential problem areas of elementary educators. *Education*, *125*(4), 615–627.
Keates, A. M., & Pearson, M. (2024). Multiple intelligences theory and expressive therapies: New counselling options for secondary school students who experience anxiety. *Journal of Psychologists and Counsellors in Schools*, *34*(1), 120–129.

Kim, J. B., Kirchhoff, M., & Whitsett, S. (2011). Expressive arts group therapy with middle-school aged children from military families. *The Arts in Psychotherapy, 38*(5), 356–362.

Knight, K., Gibson, K., & Cartwright, C. (2018). "It's like a refuge": Young people's relationships with school counsellors. *Counselling and Psychotherapy Research, 18*(4), 377–386.

Koithan, M. (2009). Introducing complementary and alternative therapies. *The Journal for Nurse Practitioners, 5*(1), 18–20.

Lahue, K., Rivera, E., & Schmidt, S. (2023). The exploration of the experience of expressive therapies in a pediatric medical setting in the COVID-19 pandemic through arts-based research. *OBM Integrative and Complementary Medicine, 8*(4), 1–24.

Lavania, C., & Ballal, D. (2025). The application of expressive art therapies for survivors of child sexual abuse. *Psychological Trauma: Theory, Research, Practice, and Policy.* Advance online publication.

Martin, D. J., Garske, J. P., & Davis, M. K. (2000). Relation of the therapeutic alliance with outcome and other variables: a meta-analytic review. *Journal of consulting and clinical psychology, 68*(3), 438–450.

Maslow, E. (1970). *Motivation and personality* (2nd ed.). Harper and Row.

Mayer, J. D., & Salovey, P. (1995). Emotional intelligence and the construction and regulation of feelings. *Applied and Preventive Psychology, 4*(3), 197–208.

McKenzie, W. (1999). Multiple intelligences survey. http://surfaquarium.com/MI/index.htm

McLeod, J. (2013). *An introduction to research in counselling and psychotherapy.* Sage Publications.

McLeod, J. (2018). *Pluralistic therapy: Distinctive features.* Routledge.

McVeigh, B. J. (2022). *The self-healing mind: Harnessing the active ingredients of psychotherapy.* Oxford University Press.

Midgley, N., Hayes, J., & Cooper, M. (2017). *Essential research findings in child and adolescents counselling and psychotherapy.* Sage.

Moran, S., Kornhaber, M., & Gardner, H. (2006). Orchestrating multiple intelligences. *Educational Leadership, 64*(1), 22–27.

Nolen, J. L. (2003). Multiple intelligences in the classroom. *Education, 124*(1), 115–119.

Norcross, J. C. (2005). The psychotherapist's own psychotherapy: Educating and developing psychologists. *American Psychologist, 60*(8), 840–850.

O'Brien, P., & Burnett, P. (2000). Counselling children using a multiple intelligence framework. *British Journal of Guidance and Counselling, 28*(3), 353–371.

Ozceker, D., Adali, B. Y., Aktas, S., Tomru, D. S., Tamay, Z., & Güler, N. (2023). Expressive arts therapy with asthmatic children: The effects of an 8-week intervention study. *Pediatrics International, 65*(1), e15452.

Pattison, S., & Harris, B. (2006). Adding value to education through improved mental health: A review of the research evidence on the effectiveness of counselling for children and young people. *Australian Educational Researcher, 33*(2), 97–122.

Pearson, M. (2003). Guidance officer and counsellor perspectives on using expressive therapies to support students. *Australian Journal of Guidance and Counselling, 13*(2), 205–224.

Pearson, M. (2011). Multiple intelligences and the therapeutic alliance: Incorporating multiple intelligence theory and practice in counselling. *European Journal of Psychotherapy & Counselling*, *13*(3), 263–278.

Pearson, M., & de Bruin, M. (2019). Counsellors as resilience guides: Ten ways that counselling support can develop resilience. *Counselling Australia*, *19*(1), 28–35.

Pearson, M., & O'Brien, P. (2012). Changing views of theory and practice in counselling: Multiple intelligences, eclecticism and the therapeutic alliance. *Psychotherapy & Counselling Journal of Australia*, *1*(1), 15–28.

Pearson, M., O'Brien, P., & Bulsara, C. (2015). A multiple intelligences approach to counseling: Enhancing alliances with a focus on strengths. *Journal of Psychotherapy Integration*, *25*(1), 128–142.

Pearson, M., & Wilson, H. (2009). *Using expressive arts to work with mind, body and emotions: Theory and practice*. Jessica Kingsley Publishers.

Pearson, M., & Wilson, H. (2024). Therapeutic relating in expressive therapies: Reflections on being with young clients. *Counselling Australia*, *1*(1), Online edition.

Polínek, M. D., & Telekyová, T. (2025). Child development in primary school through expressive therapeutic approaches. In *Conference Proceedings. The Future of Education 15th Edition, 2025.*

Poznanski, J., & McLennan, J. (2004). Theoretical orientation and the person of the therapist: An Australian study. *Psychotherapy in Australia*, *10*(3), 62–65.

Rodrigues, V., & Friedman, H. L. (2013). Transpersonal psychotherapies. In H. L. Friedman & G. Hartelius (Eds.), *The Wiley-Blackwell handbook of transpersonal psychology* (pp. 580–594). Wiley-Blackwell.

Rogers, C. R. (1951). *Client-centered therapy – Its current practice, implications and theory*. Constable.

Rogers, C. R. (1967). *On becoming a person: A therapist's view of psychotherapy*. Houghton Mifflin Company.

Shearer, C. B. (1996). *The MIDAS: Professional manual*. MI Research and Consulting, Inc.

Shepard, R., Fasko Jr, D., & Osborne, F. H. (1999). Intrapersonal intelligence: Affective factors in thinking. *Education*, *119*(4), 633–642.

Siegel, J., Iida, H., Rachlin, K., & Yount, G. (2016). Expressive arts therapy with hospitalized children: A pilot study of co-creating healing sock creatures. *Journal of Pediatric Nursing*, *31*(1), 92–98.

Siu, A. F., & Chan, A. H. (2020). Multimodal expressive arts in school counselling: A strength-based intervention program for academic underachievers in secondary schools. *Asia Pacific Journal of Counselling and Psychotherapy*, *11*(2), 139–158.

Southwell, J. (2016). Using 'expressive therapies' to treat developmental trauma and attachment problems in preschool-aged children. *Children Australia*, *41*(2), 114–125.

Swift, J. K., Callahan, J. L., Ivanovic, M., & Kominiak, N. (2013). Further examination of the psychotherapy preference effect: A meta-regression analysis. *Journal of Psychotherapy Integration*, *23*(2), 134.

Talens, P. (2024). *What is the relationship between the extent of manualised practice and 'effective' psychotherapy?* (Doctoral thesis). University of Roehampton.

Teele, S. (1992). *Teele inventory of multiple intelligences*. Sue Teele and Associates.

Visser, B. A., Ashton, M. C., & Vernon, P. A. (2006). Beyond g: Putting multiple intelligences theory to the test. *Intelligence*, *34*(5), 487–502.

Watson, J. C., & Lemon, J. C. (2011). A profile of adolescent wellness: Implications for working with a help-seeking population. *The Journal of Humanistic Counseling*, *50*(1), 70–83.

Westergaard, J. (2013). Counselling young people: Counsellors' perspectives on 'what works' – An exploratory study. *Counselling and Psychotherapy Research*, *13*(2), 98–105.

World Health Organization. (n.d.). https://www.who.int/mental_health/maternal-child/child_adolescent/en/

Zakaria, M. (2015). The efficacy of expressive arts therapy in the creation of catharsis in counselling. *Mediterranean Journal of Social Sciences*, *6*(6), 298–306.

2 Setting the Stage

Therapeutic Integration and Planning

Integration of Approaches to Counselling Children

Some of the foundations of ET – indeed as with many of the integrative therapies – lie in the early development of Western psychotherapy. The eclectic and practical choices in ET's therapeutic activities have been drawn from a wide range of theories and approaches, primarily infused with a creative arts therapies' heritage. In addition to Creative Arts Therapies, the approaches and theories that inform ET include: Person-centred Therapy, Psychodynamic Counselling, Attachment Theory, Analytic Psychology, Emotion-Focused Therapy, Cognitive and Behavioural Approaches, Gestalt Therapy, Systemic Approaches, Play Therapy, Transpersonal Psychotherapy, Focusing, Bioenergetics, as well as a few aspects of post-modern approaches.

Person-Centred Therapy

Person-centred Therapy (PCT), the humanistic approach developed by Rogers (1951), has a focus on nurturing the client's emotional needs, establishing a democratic relationship with the client and establishing who the "problem" most impacts. With its emphasis on deep listening, empowerment and collaborative problem solving, Rogers' well-researched application of empathy, unconditional positive regard and genuineness remains a core ingredient to successful outcomes at the heart of contemporary practice (Cooper, 2004).

Successful therapy with young clients relies on a person-centred approach. Rogers' (1961) early research on core elements for positive therapeutic outcomes identified genuineness as a major contributor. While PCT was proposed over eighty years ago, there is growing, recent evidence for the effectiveness of Humanistic approaches (e.g., Midgley et al., 2017). What stands out from research into PCT is the importance of empathy, unconditional positive regard and congruence within the therapeutic alliance. High levels of these attitudes have been found to lead to improved positive outcomes for a client. Alarmingly, low levels of these attitudes lead to client deterioration, and increased potential for negative outcomes for clients (Midgley et al., 2017)

DOI: 10.4324/9781003671879-2

A person-centred approach acknowledges the importance of formal knowledge, theory and repetition of particular therapeutic structures, but has as a primary focus the development of the relationship with the young client. Client-centredness means offering a wide range of possible therapeutic activities that can support growth towards improved self-image and ability to make positive choices. Through absence of judgement, positive regard within a caring therapeutic relationship, clients are empowered to choose from multiple means for reflection, communication and expression. A growth-focused attitude, as a core premise in ET, provides the means to collaborate with a client to find a way forward in each moment of therapy. From an ET perspective, the best way forward is considered the way a client prefers to reflect and express themselves so as to communicate their concerns as clearly as possible, and have experiences of feeling heard and "seen" by another.

Rogers (1961) cautioned against adopting a façade, a persona of psychological knower, or the all-knowing expert. In truth, this is rarely observed in professional counsellors whose work is centred on the mental health of young people. Young clients are unlikely to respond well if we relate to them as if we hold the all-powerful position in the dynamic. What is known is any effort to be genuine is clearly perceived by young clients and helps them begin to trust. The fundamental stance in relation to a client is our confidence that, with support, they can find their way, tap into internal resources and connect with an intrinsic positive growth trajectory.

Psychodynamic Counselling

The psychodynamic approach, built on the psychoanalytic work of Freud and Klein, views problems as having a source in the past, and at times in the unconscious. This approach aims to release emotional energy connected to past anxieties. Psychodynamic therapists attempt to help clients identify patterns in their emotions, thoughts and beliefs as a process of developing greater awareness of their current ways of interpersonal interaction. The origins of these patterns are often found in a client's childhood experiences. Psychodynamic theory holds that early life experiences are extremely influential in the psychological development and functioning of an adult (Jacobs, 1988).

What characterises a psychodynamic approach is a belief in the power of forgotten experiences and the use of therapeutic relationships to enable a deeper connection with self. Central to the effectiveness of the therapy process is a premise that the working alliance established with a client is the conduit through which issues of endings, transference and countertransference are explored and worked through (Hetherington, 1999). A psychodynamic approach conceptualises that past experiences influence present choices, moods and behaviours, and suggests that, at times, recall, resolution, release and understanding of earlier experiences are essential for therapeutic success. Creative arts modalities have proven to be highly effective in supporting clients to concretise memories, feelings, reactions, that have been implicit or forgotten.

Adolescents can be puzzled by their behaviours, which can lead to the opposite response to what they need. The psychodynamic framework can be most helpful in these cases. For example, timeline work that utilises worksheets, sketches, or arrangements of miniatures can support an understanding of times and places where something happened, or should have happened; times and places that have impacted on growth, progress and happiness. The "Thinking About My LIfe" activity (page 219) has been found particularly useful for making links across stages of life, illuminating past events that contributed to current reactivity.

With a basis adapted from a psychodynamic perspective, expressive therapists are sensitive to clients' attachment history and needs. This is important because of the links between what fuels emotional reactivity and unprocessed or incomplete emotions. From this perspective, reliving and processing "unfinished business" can become – this time round with non-judgemental support – a major focus. It can be ideal therefore, when the time is right, to assist clients in acknowledging feelings, exploring and embracing a softening of defensive behaviours.

We know that the body, mind and feelings work as a whole. This means that what is not acknowledged or expressed becomes held and experienced internally as negative. Muscular tension links the body to psychological holding. Long-term tension creates fertile ground for disruptive or destructive thoughts. Eventually, those can be expressed as unproductive, negative behaviours. Providing activities that enhance a young client's somatic, emotional and cognitive awareness and reduce mechanisms that maintain physical holding can lead to more emotional balance and a decrease in reactive behaviours. Reducing experiential avoidance, while temporarily uncomfortable, enables resolution of the past and promotes openness to positivity and creativity. With resolution comes physical relaxation and greater capacity to relate more easily with others in the outer world.

Though unresolved emotion may seem invisible, and associated memories appear forgotten, the influence on behaviour continues. Bringing what is not resolved to awareness is the first step in reducing influence on how a young person lives. Release of frustrations and stresses may be sufficient for some child clients to recover positive functioning. Full resolution of more challenging background issues may need to wait until adulthood. In the context of a safe, positive therapeutic alliance, young clients can and do make it clear when they feel there has been sufficient turning towards the past, reviewing what has happened, or exploration and expression of unpleasant experiences.

Young clients whose life experiences have left an indelible legacy of distance from their sense of worth, their sense of being a resilient person, can benefit from dealing directly with past issues. There can also be a storehouse of forgotten positive qualities, positive feelings and memories, that remain overshadowed or inactive. This is particularly so when a family culture may be predominantly problem-focused, and even more so when there is a legacy of trauma. So, while being attentive to unfinished business may be the core of psychodynamically focused work, bringing forgotten positive traits and experiences to awareness can strengthen a sense of self. Indeed, having an early focus on discerning strengths and positive traits is highly recommended.

Attachment Theory

John Bowlby's Attachment Theory (Holmes, 2014) suggests that therapists contribute to an experience of secure attachment and support the development of a more secure sense of the world for a client. Behavioural problems traced to attachment issues are likely to surface in the client-therapist relationship (Pearce & Pezzot-Pearce, 1994). Therapists can interact in a way that can soothe these concerns. Essentially, regular, ongoing support allows young clients to participate in the session and the therapeutic relationship at their own pace.

Bosmans (2016) described the way enhancing parent-child attachment can make significant increases in otherwise moderate CBT outcomes. This author does not, however, describe the role of the therapist as provider of attachment security. Remaining non-reactive when attempts at connection are rejected by the client, and conveying acceptance – verbally or non-verbally – contributes to neural development in the brain's attachment area (Schore, 2000). This supports a client to establish a more secure, regulated and resilient outlook. For counsellors, understanding how a client's "internal working model" (Bretherton, 1999) perceives self and the world helps make sense of client behaviour that otherwise could appear to sabotage hoped-for outcomes.

Analytic Psychology

Jung's Analytic Psychology (Samuels, 2003) invites us to consider how unconscious or implicit memory may have more influence than conscious or explicit intent. This concept is one supported by findings from neuroscience research (e.g., Cappas et al., 2005). There is an intrinsic movement in the human psyche towards healing, wholeness and differentiation, a movement Jung named "individuation". While Jung and his colleagues focused on the later stages of this process, the early stages required resolution of complexes, neuroses and other negative outcomes from early life. This concept calls therapists to explore ways to understand and cooperate with this inherent tendency, and interpret client behaviours from this perspective.

Jung explored the way working with dreams and symbols within dreams had the potential to provide self-understanding. Symbols are regarded as the language of the unconscious, and unconscious or implicit memory functions symbolically (Rothschild, 2000). Dream images, metaphors and miniatures are widely used in ET to assist in deeper self-understanding, in the self-reflection process, as well as self-expression, emotional processing and integration. For clients in recovery from trauma, tolerating symbol work (with miniatures) can contribute to experience by creating safe links between implicit and explicit experiences.

Emotion-Focused Therapy

Emotion-Focused Therapy (EFT) founders Greenberg (2004) and Johnson (2018) argue for the central role of emotion in psychotherapeutic change. Their work provided a revised orientation of the relationship between cognition and emotion. EFT is an integrative, empirically based approach, based on methods designed to help people accept, express, regulate, make sense of and transform emotion. This approach proposes that working through emotion is a necessary step prior to enhanced cognitive clarity or understanding behavioural change. In general, after accessing, accepting and experiencing emotion, clients are guided to review and understand their experiences. Greenberg clearly recommends that emotion "schemes", or patterns of emotion, are activated within the safety of a positive therapeutic relationship, providing potential for resolution. He cites empirical support for the effectiveness of a range of emotionally focused intervention strategies (Greenberg, 2004). In ET practice, working with emotion is offered as part of Stage 3 of a 5 Stage Model. Safe, supported processing of emotions brings capacity for clients to integrate a more positive view of themselves. Greenberg notes: "Most fundamentally, emotions tell us what is important to us in a situation and thus act as a guide to what we need or want. This, in turn, helps us to figure out what actions are appropriate" (https://www.yorku.ca/health/eft/ n.d.).

Emotion-focused processes, developed as part of the repertoire of ET techniques, subscribe to the principles Greenberg and Johnson argue for in EFT. Transition through the stages of emotion-focused work is effectively supported by numerous ET modalities (see more in Chapter 7).

Cognitive and Behavioural Approaches

Cognitive and behavioural approaches became combined into a seemingly ever-expanding integration of CBT (Rachman, 2015). At its inception, CBT combined models and strategies tied together by the aim to review and revise habitual thoughts and behaviours. Since its inception, this approach has become more eclectic. Contemporary CBT practice incorporates activities that take into account a client's physiological, psychological and emotional needs.

The ET focus on first attending to being heard and emotional resolution can bring the client to a readiness to address behaviour. The ET Five-Stage Model (see pages 36 to 46) addresses behaviour, behavioural planning, discussion of core beliefs and identification of potential changes in behaviour and self-talk in Stage 5, the final stage.

Behaviourist approaches are based on the premise that behaviour is learned and can therefore be unlearned – a concept developed from animal-based research by B. F. Skinner (Catania & Harnad, 1988). Behavioural change involved the application of positive and negative reinforcement. Criticism of the autocratic application of therapy tasks (Porter, 2020) generated some questions about long-term efficacy. Development of client awareness of influences on, and consequences of, their behaviour can however be useful. To attend solely to behaviour change, without attending to underlying motivations, can be counter-productive in terms of overall wellbeing for a child client. ET activities for reflection on behaviour change are offered in session Stage 5 (see page 46).

Cognitive Therapy aims to identify and revise beliefs, attitudes, self-talk and thinking patterns that underlie negative acting-out behaviours, with a focus on adjustment of dysfunctional thinking. Critics of a purely cognitive approach (e.g., Hammack, 2003; Rachman, 1993) suggest that cognitive changes may be short-lived if emotional concerns remain unaddressed. The theory underlying cognitive therapy may therefore be incompatible with a postmodern perspective on the human condition.

To support a young client, identifying unhelpful beliefs and thinking patterns may be productive. ET therapeutic writing activities can explore and expand self-concepts; for example, see page 108 and 109. ET also uses non-cognitive means to help a client reach cognitive clarity. For example, arrangements of miniatures, followed by discussion, are one way to distinguish between behaviours and values.

Mindfulness and creative arts activities have been combined into contemporary CBT practice. Using ET activities, the contemporary functional analysis process (Hayes & O'Brien, 1990), at the heart of CBT practice, can be more easily and effectively explored. Both ET and CBT aim to broaden client capacity for self-awareness. Both ET and CBT agree that enhanced self-awareness will likely lead to increased capacity for more productive behaviour choices.

Gestalt Therapy

One of the main founders of Gestalt Therapy, Fritz Perls, held a keen interest in what he believed to be a process of reclamation of alienated parts of self (Perls, 1969). One of Perls' main psychotherapeutic methods was inviting clients to explore dream symbols using a role-play technique, developed from drama training. From Gestalt Therapy comes the now widely used ET role-play activity, developed in 1988 by Pearson and Nolan (2004), that supports clients reclaim a previously disowned positive sense of self, energy, feelings and strengths.

Perls' concept of movement of issues between the foreground and background in the psyche suggests that we listen to clients' narratives to ascertain what might be standing out to them, in addition to what seems to be in the foreground to us. Some approaches train therapists to offer feedback to a client on what was observed in behaviours, statements, or even artefacts created in session. A preferred therapeutic stance in ET is to ask the client what they notice, leading to greater understanding of their unique perspective or insight.

Oaklander's (1978) gestalt-oriented Play Therapy activities also provided inspiration for the development of ET. Her direct encouragement for an early ET text (Pearson & Nolan, 2004) supported the ongoing evolution of our approach to ET. Frankel (1998) pointed out that children may not be able to negotiate adults' "world of words", but are "fluent at communicating through action" (p. 173). It is in providing action for young clients that Oaklander, and the traditional play therapists, for example Axline (1947), show as a way forward for work with young clients who may prefer not to engage directly with us, or to communicate through language.

Systemic Approaches

Therapies created for use with distressed families and couples (e.g., Johnson, 2018; Minuchin, 2014) aim at improvement in the relationship between family members and partners. This is particularly so between an "identified client" and their family, as well as within wider social networks. Looking beyond the individual, intrapsychic exploration of a psychodynamic approach, systemic therapists look for ways to improve interpersonal interactions and bring to light any interactions that maintain relational challenges.

A client's view of their lived context can be identified, explored and communicated well with ET activities. Expressing family dynamics through arranging miniatures in combination with sketching and integrative discussion can reveal issues to be addressed within a family. Arranging and manipulating the miniatures can help a client gain clarity about interpersonal dynamics and provide a guide to develop expressive reciprocal interactions that improve relational connection.

ET contributes positively to family therapy approaches. There is a long history of established thought that privileges verbal communication. "Action methods" (Wiener & Oxford, 2003) have, however, been offered in supporting families since the 1960s. Expressive Therapies (ET) extends those action methods through use of engaging and non-threatening creative arts activities.

Family sessions can be highly charged. It makes sense, therefore, to include interventions that engage self-reflection, relational exploration, and appropriate expression of emotions that aim to generate insight on interpersonal dynamics and enhanced empathy and a shared understanding. Experiential, engaged, emotional and somatic understanding can soften interpersonal defensiveness and motivate the development of revised positively aligned interactions.

A range of creative arts therapists have brought to family therapy the use of visual art, dance, psychodrama, multimodal play and music (Wiener & Oxford, 2003). Expressive approaches mean family members engage in a more direct relational experience – understanding patterns of defence. Evoking increased empathy along with cognitive and emotional shifts creates new relational possibilities (Haley, 1976; Minuchin, 1974). ET activities provide a therapist with a first-hand view of verbal and nonverbal communications of family members. In an individual session, ET supports client exploration of emotion-laden family dynamics.

A child client may be unable to express – to parents or to the therapist – beliefs and feelings they have about what is going on in the family. Permission to represent the family in symbolic form, without the need to be explicit, means reduced distress about disclosure and loyalty. The element of play has been used in family therapy for over 30 years. Pioneers in family therapy, such as Whitaker and Keith (1981) believed that play is ideally an integral part of family therapy.

Play Therapy

Play Therapy has a long history and includes approaches that are either undirected (e.g., Axline, 1989) or directed (e.g., Booth & Jernberg, 2009). Undirected, or non-directive (Ahuja & Saha, 2016), Play Therapy provides opportunities for spontaneous expression, free choice and non-verbal engagement and communication through the use of a large range of media in a way similar to ET. While Play Therapy has been found to be effective with a broad range of ages, undirected, or "non-directive" Play Therapy would be particularly useful for clients under the age of six, who, in general, are less interested in following stepped or directed activities.

With the therapist's witnessing presence a major contributor, Play Therapy allows internal conflicts to be acted out in ways that can lead to resolution. This technique operates on a foundation of trust that a client has the ability to naturally work through issues, to vent, create and "re-story" through spontaneous play. Directed Play Therapy, for example, Theraplay (Booth & Jernberg, 2009), resembles to some extent some of the structured ET activities that guide a client through steps and stages of an outcome-oriented experiential activity.

Transpersonal Psychotherapy

Jung has been considered to be one of the forerunners of a transpersonal perspective within therapy (Grof, 1998; Vaughan, 2012), particularly through his concept of a collective unconscious. Like transpersonal psychologists, Jung considered that understanding or accessing the spiritual dimension may be essential for growth and healing.

Grof's conceptualisation of Transpersonal Psychology includes awareness of the impact of difficult perinatal (around the birth) experiences. Grof's ideas suggest a trauma-informed blueprint that, unaddressed, can influence behaviour patterns and ultimately shape personality. Perinatal stresses cannot normally be accessed or resolved through talk and reliance on cognition. Acknowledgement of pre-verbal stressors suggests that therapists support clients to play out internal stresses in physical, emotional, as well as symbolic, ways. When a therapist remains curious and open to a transpersonal dimension of the psyche, this openness may allow young clients to share perspectives, stories or dreams that seem outside the parameters of what is experienced in everyday life.

In a research project with 16 to 17 year-olds, themes of "conscious interactions, compassion/generosity, and aspiring for beauty/wisdom" were found to be most important (Bussing et al., 2010). Youth futures researchers have linked a loss of meaning and purpose to the contemporary secular societal context in which young people experience a sense of a spiritual vacuum within society (Gidley, 2005). This suggests when a searching or curious nature can be met with support, with "conscious interactions, compassion and generosity". Sadly, some evidence suggests students would likely be discouraged from exploring or expressing spiritual beliefs and questions in some school settings (Schwarz, 2013). Schwarz (2013) also found that spirituality was an aspect of students' identities that school counsellors reported avoiding in their work.

From discoveries of the psychotherapeutic process of holotropic breathwork (Grof et al., 2010), comes the use of breath to expand contact with the depths of the psyche and allow what has been called the "inner healer" to guide a therapeutic process. Many approaches to physical and mental health use breath (Victoria & Caldwell, 2013). In particular the use of breath is central in body-oriented psychotherapy. The well-documented (Victoria & Caldwell, 2013) positive physical effects of focused and expanded breathing can have "a profound influence on psychological wellbeing, particularly in the areas of mood, reduction of negative emotion, and an increase in positive emotion, emotional regulation and the capacity for social engagement" (Victoria & Caldwell, 2013, p. 217). Breath in ET is used as an invitation to a client to turn inward and explore their own knowing. ET breathing processes make it more possible for a client to become aware of their emotional life. ET incorporates multiple ways to encourage young clients to take deeper breaths, to play with breath, and to role-play creatures that display lots of breath, for example, fire-breathing dragons, whales, dogs panting after a run (See more on this page 151).

Focusing

From experiential developments in psychotherapy, (e.g., Gendlin, 1999) comes the extensive use in ET of supporting clients in mindfulness-oriented "tuning-in"; allowing time and attention to be given to connect internally with body sensations, emotions, energetic states and, of course, repeating thought patterns. Time for internal focus generates increased capacity for self-awareness. This in turn enables a client to recognise and share experiences that may guide the focus of a session. In addition, what is experienced may provide guidance for the client's behaviour in daily life. In Gendlin's approach, developed in the 1950s, in collaboration with Carl Rogers, the main concepts are accessing bodily felt sense, allowing fresh descriptions to emerge from this experience, and integrating small, almost implicit steps of change (Hendricks, 2007).

Mindfulness and focusing-oriented activities that mirror Gendlin's approach have always been central in the evolution of ET. Gendlin's clients were guided to "pay attention to what is, at first, a vague yet persistent, bodily felt sense of some problem or situation. Clients pause, grope for words to get at this sense, and often create a metaphor to describe it. When they find words or an image that "gets it exactly", there is a felt relief and sense of meaning and movement" (Hendricks, 2007, p. 271). This description of the therapeutic process through focusing lends weight to the ever-present invitation ET counsellors offer: To tune in, and see what the client notices internally, so that their awareness can expand leading to more intentional relating with self and the world.

For more on the ET use of Body Focus activities see page 139.

Bioenergetics

Alexander Lowen's (1977/2012) bioenergetic exercises were based on principles for psychotherapy outlined by Wilhelm Reich. Bioenergetics are experiential, emotional, physical and energetic release activities that when introduced added further depth to Western therapy. This approach sits comfortably in the field of somatic psychotherapy. The importance of the flow of bioenergy is regarded by the creators of bioenergetics as essential for emotional and mental health. ET bioenergetic games and activities, which are essentially child-friendly adaptations of exercises developed for adult clients, have been based on the observation that young clients have needed to contain their difficult experiences. This results in muscular tension and disconnection from emotion. Through engaging in bioenergetic games, young clients' contact with their bodily and emotional experience is enhanced to support physical relaxation.

Movement or kinaesthetic activities, from the repertoire of ET activities, such as energy release or bioenergetic exercises, are useful to reduce chronic body tension (see more on this page 154). In his writings, Reich referred to chronic tension as "body armouring". Armouring is believed to interrupt natural emotional and energetic flow. Reich (1933/1980) argued that an important step towards mental health was to acknowledge, address and process negatively geared emotions such as anger and even hate, and that this process required somatic expression of affect. Eliciting catharsis was core in Reich's work, as was the case in Freud's early work. However, catharsis appeared to fall from mainstream Western psychology, partly due to Freud's abandonment of it (Nichols & Efran, 1985). Unpopularity of catharsis in a therapy setting may in part be due to an important, but missing element of time for emotional and cognitive integration, after emotional expression. Perhaps integration was not significant or fully understood or applied at that time. The result has been a limited or marred evidence base for cathartic approaches (more on this on page 174).

Post-Modern Approaches

Solution-Focused Brief Therapy (SFBT) (De Shazer & Berg, 1997) promotes a cognitive focus on activating strengths and looking beyond problems to solutions. Solution-focused approaches guide a therapist to questions such as: *What do you do that works? Could you do more of that?* To establish a practical vision of a better future, they often ask what has become known as the "miracle question", a version of: *If – tomorrow morning – all the problems were gone, what would that look like?* The valuable components of SFBT help create an image of a problem-free future in the belief that clients would then be motivated to develop clearer goals. An expressive therapist offers the use of art and arranging miniatures as ways to symbolise new and emerging images of the future (more on this on page 87).

The main criticisms of SFBT (e.g., Walker et al., 2021) are that practitioners may overlook problems completely or attempt to bypass the often challenging task of working with difficult emotions. The risk of working in an entirely cognitive way, without reference to emotion or somatic experience, is generally a vision of something better, but without a pathway to attain it.

Narrative Therapy (NT) (White, 2003) offers an approach for restructuring life stories. The impetus is to move aside from sustained problem focus. NT can shed light on the way clients tell themselves and others a story that becomes a basis for their sense of self, for relating and for high or low optimism. Central to NT is the deliberate task of re-storying. The process of re-storying is often evoked organically through engagement with ET art-making and therapeutic writing modalities. Additionally, through the creation and narration of arrangements of miniatures, either in a sandtray or on a desk or table, presents a new image – or story – of self and life. Enhanced resilience and increased motivation to engage in therapy and everyday living emerge.

Creative Arts Therapies

ET has drawn extensively from the creative arts therapy traditions. These traditions have long histories, and we appreciate the gifts of the pioneers of each modality, for example art therapy (Naumburg, 1958), sandplay therapy (Kalff, 2003) – [evolved from Lowenfeld's *World Technique* (1950)] – music therapy (Biley, 1999; Corning, 1912), poetry therapy (Jaskoski, 1980), movement and dance therapy, and drama therapy (Austin, 1917; Moreno, 1947/2010). These therapies have been applied within a diverse number of theoretical frameworks and make for an integrated approach in ET.

Expressive Therapies

ET has evolved from an integration of a range of methods, concepts and theories. The application of ET can support clients in addressing beliefs, patterns of thinking and behavioural habits, in an indirect way that is empowering for young clients. In ET, having multiple ways to symbolically express internal experiences and process emotions leads to emotional resolution, followed up with integration strategies and forward planning.

ET is pluralistic. It offers multiple modes for conducting therapy in response to client preferences and capacities. See more on pluralism on page 6. A creative arts-based collation of activities and approaches, ET has a central focus of processing emotion (Pearson & Wilson, 2009). Expressive therapists prize flexibility, drawing the most relevant therapeutic stance or activities from a range of approaches to offer what is most suitable for each client in each session.

The ET Five-Stage Model for Planning Sessions

The dance between being ready, doing our homework, preparing for what might be most helpful for clients, vs. being attentive, in the moment, spontaneous, collaborative and client-led, will always be with us. After doing our best to plan for an individual client, we hold that plan lightly. We remain open to what is most needed in any moment of a session.

To define exactly how a session will progress or to prescribe a certain progression through the counselling process is not possible. However, we have developed a five-stage ET session model as a basic guide to identify a potential rational flow of therapeutic intentions. Each client moves in a unique and highly individualised way through the issues that catalysed their therapeutic journey. It is helpful to remember our clients are not pieces of a jigsaw to be re-arranged, or crosswords to complete. The range and exact nature of issues to be addressed may not be evident when clients first enter therapy. The client arrives as a type of container and therapy is the process that provides both containment and forward movement with clearing the "container". Our effort to conceptualise the direction of therapy is as important in our preparation as our capacity to understand their intentions for seeking therapy. Autonomy, however, means a client may seek to address one current-day topic only and not "dig" deeper.

From a person-centred perspective, the focus always remains on the young client and what they need, and the pace they determine therapy is to move. ET stresses the importance of discovering the young person's preference for the way the therapeutic work is conducted. Despite the emphasis on fluidity and flexibility in responding to client needs, the five-stage model gives the therapist an outline of what they might prepare to offer as sessions progress.

Diagram 1 depicts our Five-Stage Model, which includes an optional sixth stage. That sixth stage provides for the inclusion of homework and/or self-care strategies that may assist the client in processing session contents and managing life. Each of these stages will be discussed in detail. The first five stages are the essence of the model, homework remains optional, and should not be offered at every session. While presented here in a linear fashion, in practice the stages remain flexible, circular and recursive.

Summary of the ET Five-Stage Model

1. Who are we? Breaking the ice, building safety and rapport, early assessment and learning about the client.
2. Turning within: Building self-awareness, opening to self-understanding.
3. Expression: Processing emotion.
4. Integration: Cooling down and making sense of session experiences.
5. The way forward: Support for planning, problem-solving, strategy formulation and creativity.

Optional Homework and Self-Care.

This model does not suggest that each stage would take only one session. What is represented is a pared-down version of complexities that become apparent in ET. It should be noted that the behavioural aspects of therapy are placed in Stage 5, after there is opportunity to resolve emotions that may have been impacting behaviour. A client may move through these stages in rapid succession, or may require extended time as they oscillate between Stages 2 and 3 until emotional distress feels dissipated and emotionally charged memories are integrated into balanced functioning. Stages 1, 4 and 5 are non-negotiable; the need to include these in our sessions remains constant, making these three stages a standard part of any ET session.

We are intensely interested and attentive to relationship development and its ongoing unfolding (Stage 1) regardless of the number of sessions. Of course, there are some clients who may prefer to spend much time establishing the safety of Stage 1. Sometimes activities relating to Stage 2 may be sufficient to help a client resolve distress and identify what they want. Most often, some connection with, and expression of, troubling emotion will be necessary for resolution. After emotion expression, it is critical to allow time for the client to integrate, to return to a more regulated state, and make meaning of their experience (Stage 4). Cognitive engagement in meaning-making is usually central to integration and moving forward (Stage 5).

Initial ET sessions are likely, as is the case with most therapeutic approaches, to focus on Stage 1: Breaking the ice. Each client needs to feel heard, and their distress recognised and validated. This means Stage 1 may extend over several sessions, depending on the intention of a client and their readiness, or ability, to trust and develop rapport. ET activities would still be used in sessions throughout this Stage. It goes without saying that Stages 4 and 5 would be integral to a client's wellbeing as we complete each session, as well as final sessions. We operate from the perspective that a client is working with us towards completion within each session, within a larger field of moving towards more harmonious functioning.

In practice, the ET 5-Stage model is not linear, even though there is a recognisable pattern and progression through each stage (e.g., Stage 2 does not need to be "completed" before engagement in Stage 3). Sometimes a few sessions can bring a positive result and be a valuable asset for loosening the "log jam" of life's challenges. There are times when a child or adolescent arrives for a session with their emotional state clearly activated, sometimes with little capacity for containment. Emotions may be highly active and even dysregulated. This means the young person is likely to enter the session at Stage 3 without time for Stages 1 and 2. In this case, significant time would likely be needed for Stage 4. Again, as with every aspect of applying ET activities, principles and relationships, responding in this situation with flexibility is crucial.

Nancy, a 13-year-old girl, arrived for her first counselling session as a mandated client. Nancy refused to speak or look at me (HW) for the entire session time. (I never asked her to look at me or to speak – we simply sat together in silence with a few words from me at the start and end of the session). One week later, our second session was, however, very different, with Nancy arriving at the session in a heightened angry state as a result of an incident at school. Without referring to last week's resistance, Nancy responded without question to a suggestion she use crayons and paper to depict that anger and frustration. From those images, she moved without prompting to creating an image that reflected the desire to vent her rage over the insult in the classroom. Neither the first nor second session afforded time to deliberately build rapport, to explore how we would navigate our time together, or to gradually introduce her to ET resources and techniques. Nancy's comments after expending energy with crayons at the close of our second session were clear. She stated that no one had ever let her draw her anger before, but it was "really cool" to do so; she felt much calmer now; and with a tentative voice, asked was she always allowed to draw how she felt when in session with me.

Stage 1: Who Are We?

Breaking the Ice/Building Safety and Rapport/Early Assessment and Learning More about the Client

Building rapport is central to this first stage. During this time, the therapist also undertakes early observational assessment. At the start, our role is to hear the narratives that are troubling the young person. Patient attention to what is said means we come to understand a client's ways of thinking and behaving, adopted as an attempt to find relief from what is causing disruption. We learn more about their feelings about relationships within the world they inhabit. We may learn something about their attachment history. While systematic assessments, including risk assessments, are mandated in many practices, there is a challenge that these can generate caution, alienation and even be somewhat counter-productive. Learning about a client at depth takes time and trust.

Importantly, this first stage aims to facilitate foundational trust in the counsellor. Their first introduction to the therapist, the consulting room and the tools for ET activities could be both welcome relief or may come as a total surprise. Young people are, in general, mandated in some way, not the ones making an appointment. Someone else has decided there is a problem and made contact. That is, unless of course, the young person is able to self-refer.

Recommendations for the first stage of a session:

- Time for a client to develop trust in you, the setting and the therapeutic activities.
- Address their perception of why they think they have come, or been sent, to counselling.
- Provide some age-appropriate framework or rationale for counselling, and options for engagement activities.
- Accept the client as they are; hear their story without judgement or interpretation.
- Assist them to develop trust in themselves and create language with which they can articulate hunches, inclinations, as well as (therapeutic) preferences, needs and wants.
- Allow apprehension, resistance or anxiety about counselling to come forward and, if needed, be discussed and addressed before moving forward.
- Set clear boundaries for engagement in counselling. For example, clarify differences between what is welcomed in the freedom of the consulting room, and how this differs from what is welcome in other contexts.
- Invite the young person to talk about themselves and their family; use ET activities to gently explore hopes and intentions they have (if any) for their sessions, and a direction they want to move, e.g., use of miniatures, visual art symbolising thoughts and feelings, sentence starters, etc.
- Offer some ways for them to contact hopefulness, and open to recognition of internal resources and strength – e.g., *My Favourite Toy* (see page 54).

Stage 2: Turning Within

Building Self-Awareness, Opening to Self-Understanding

In this stage, we would hope the outcomes of Stage 1 discussions and activities have resulted in a willingness to turn the spotlight from external events, problems and challenges to include internal experiences. Externalising problems to minimise shame and self-blame can be an aim for Stage 2, through metaphor, artwork, miniature selection, etc. This second stage is not about making the client take responsibility, or being accountable, or somehow realising the problem may have a source inside themselves. This stage is to allow time and provide activities that activate interest in themselves and how they feel and think, and be catalysts for becoming willing clients. It may be a time when a client becomes willing to say more about what they want from counselling.

For the client who has experienced trauma, working at a gentle, slow pace is important. Working at a slow pace is much less threatening or potentially damaging than moving quickly forward and risking overwhelm or, in the worst-case scenario, re-traumatisation. Ongoing assessment is also crucial here: Is the young person ready to turn their attention towards internal processes? What evidence is there to help understand how the child or adolescent handles anxiety-laden issues? Are there any significant issues that might be missed if we move too quickly? This stage opens a time of exploration in which our attention is on the young person's internal functioning.

A range of ET processes could be introduced that help the young person discern their preference for how the sessions unfold. For instance, do they prefer drawing, music, movement, visualisations or talking? Discovery of their preferred approach to "working" will also enable identification of their preferred intelligence. Stage 2 would be the time when a short survey based on Gardner's (2006) construct of multiple intelligences could prove useful in selecting modalities that suit the client. The multiple intelligences identified from Gardner's work, and their relevance to counselling, are discussed in detail from page 8.

Our role is to accept the client as they are and convey that acceptance. During this stage, the ET tools of most assistance to facilitate the development of self-awareness and self-understanding are:

- Therapeutic Writing – e.g., responding to Sentence Starters – see Figure 2.1 and activity on page 41;
- Role-play activities using the client's selection of a positive symbol/figurine/toy;
- Developing somatic-awareness, focusing, using body outlines – see Figures 2.2 and 2.3; and activity on page 141;
- Symbol work as a catalyst to support telling their story – see Figure 2.4 and activity on page 75;

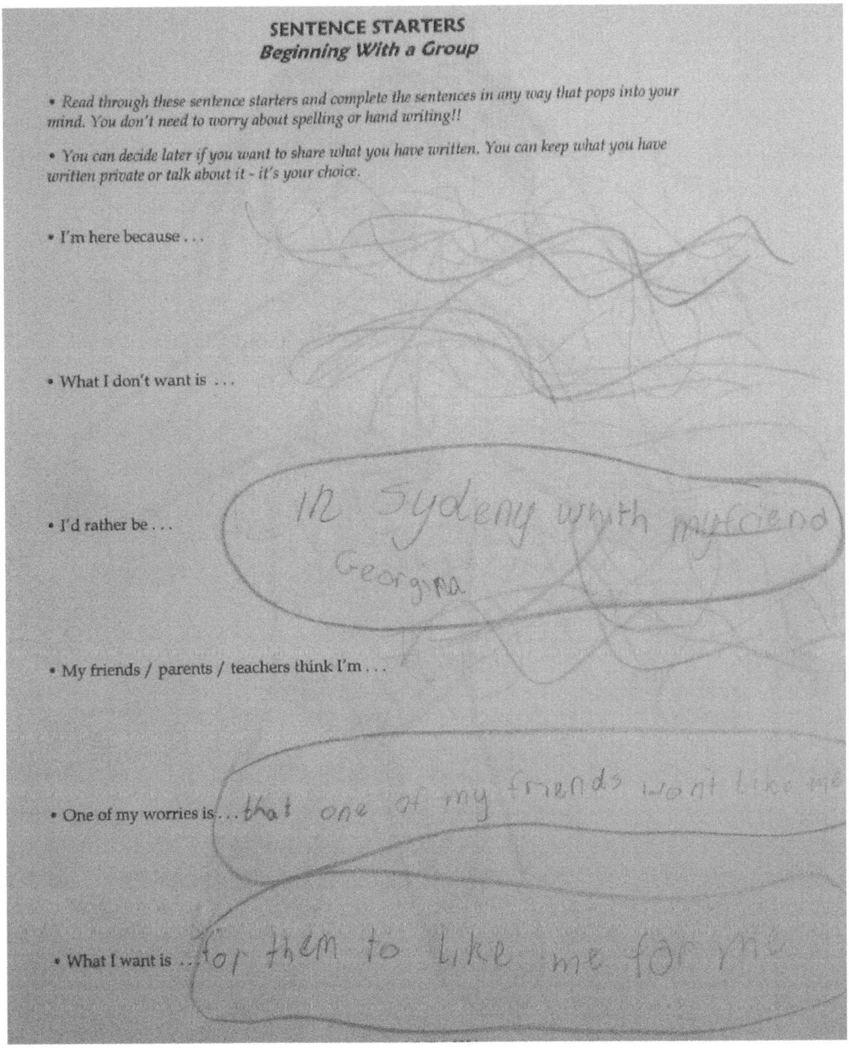

SENTENCE STARTERS
Beginning With a Group

- *Read through these sentence starters and complete the sentences in any way that pops into your mind. You don't need to worry about spelling or hand writing!!*
- *You can decide later if you want to share what you have written. You can keep what you have written private or talk about it - it's your choice.*

- I'm here because . . .
- What I don't want is . . .
- I'd rather be . . . in Sydeny whith myfriend Georgina
- My friends / parents / teachers think I'm . . .
- One of my worries is . . . that one of my friends wont like me
- What I want is . . . for them to like me for me

Figure 2.1 Responding to sentence starters.

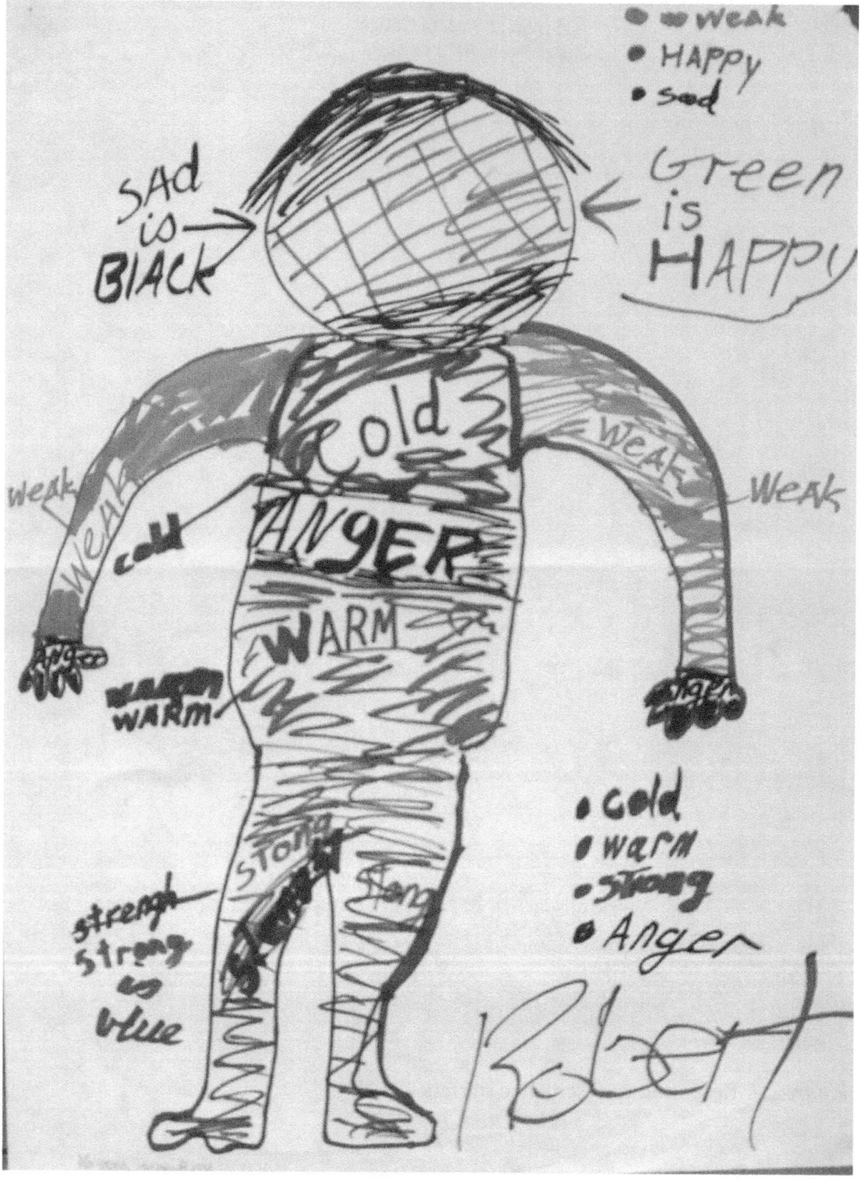

Figure 2.2 Body outline – 16-year-old male.

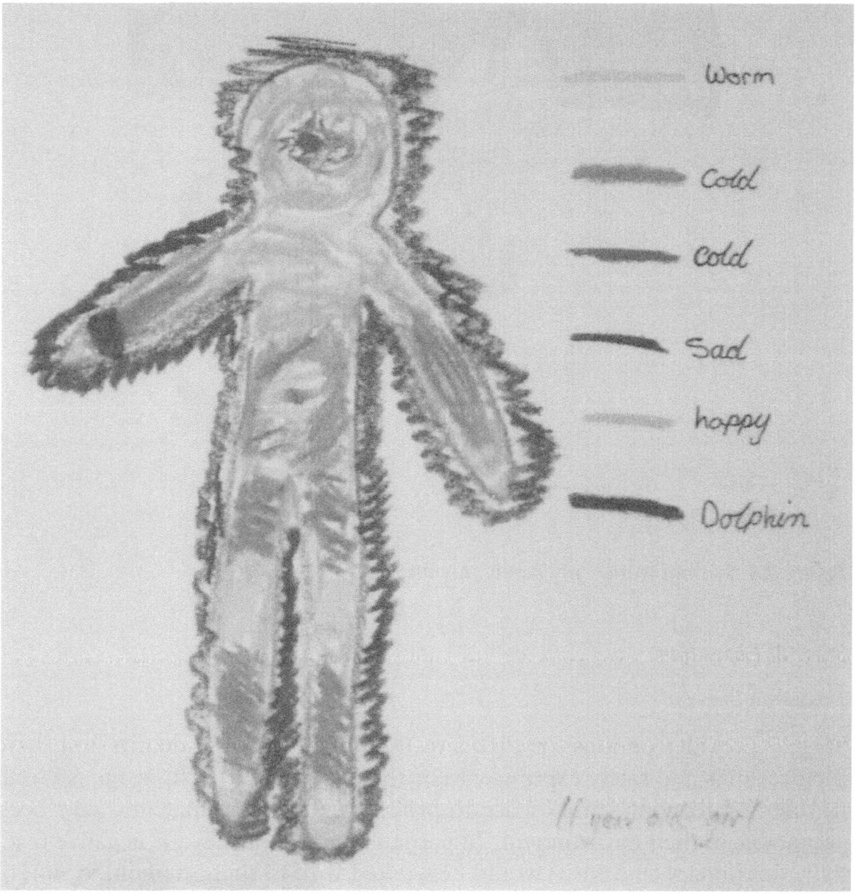

Figure 2.3 Body outline – 11 year old female.

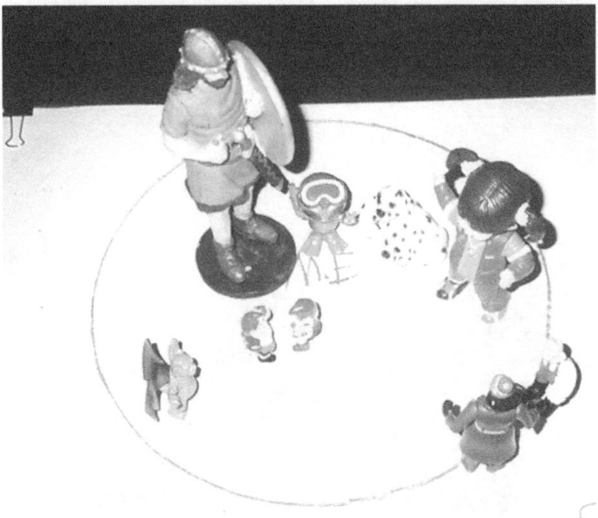

Figure 2.4 Symbol work – my family, my life.

Stage 3: Expression

Processing Emotion

Stage 3 provides options for clients to make contact with, identify and share their feelings and safely express or vent them (if needed). This stage is useful to offer a safe, confidential space to process feelings that may not have been acceptable in their environment. In particular, any tendency for negative reactivity (secondary emotions) would be worked with to support identification of the sources or starting points (primary emotions), and reduction of emotional "charge". Initiating Stage 3 is preceded by stabilising strong, positive rapport and reminders on boundaries.

Using the EFT concept of primary and secondary emotion, the young client can be supported to explore their experience of layers of emotion. Stage 3 can guide attention to any heightened reactivity, or secondary emotions, allowing these to process, enabling contact with underlying primary emotions. This "working through" of reactive emotion and underlying vulnerability can be supported through the use of:

- Process drawing and process writing (drawing and writing as spontaneous venting rather than as a planned creation) – see page 71;
- Bioenergetic games as a way to support the reduction of both physical and emotional stress – see page 152;
- Energy release games, intended for younger children, to dissipate frustrations that can drive acting-out, e.g., dramatic animal role-plays – see page 189;

- Activities to activate and work through difficult feelings, through expression with imaginary encounters. This process directs reactive thoughts and feelings, with either word, sound or movement, towards an image or objects chosen as "stand ins" for systems, people, groups or institutions. Examples of these would be:
  - Role-play of powerful animals, with use of movements and sounds to express reactions, with a focus on symbolic release – see page 189;
  - Imagine the source of reactivity as a spot on the wall and directing reactive thoughts and feelings towards it – see page 190;
  - Draw a face, or select a miniature(s) from the symbol shelves to represent the source of reactions – see page 186 and 192;
  - Imagine "other" sitting opposite and speak out emerging feelings towards the other.

At this stage, the resolution of reactivity can lead to more balanced, flexible future responses to others in their environment. If working in Stage 3, it is essential to make time for Stage 4.

Stage 4: Integration

Cooling Down and Making Sense of Experiences

If engaging with activities from Stage 3 it is vital to immediately follow up with an integration stage activity, to move towards balance and closure. Integration involves balancing right hemisphere functioning with left, heart with head, as well as allowing time for emotional arousal to dissipate. Another important component of Stage 4 is that it allows for the reabsorption of adrenaline that was released into the body in response to the stress of emotional confrontation. Reabsorption rates vary and can be influenced by the presence of past trauma, can take from 5 to 10 minutes, or longer, depending on the degree of shock or trauma the person has experienced. The primary aim is to re-confirm that the therapeutic relationship is trustworthy and safe, that the pace of therapy is directed by the client, and that there is a "safe haven" for refuge within the consulting room and, most importantly, inside themselves.

Moving towards a state of understanding and balance, as the client prepares to exit the session, can be supported through:

- Time for the client to discuss their experience of the activities.
- Reflective and completion writing – see page 102.
- Completion art – e.g., mandala drawing or other forms – see page 72.
- Movement – walking and cushion games.
- Rest, relaxation and visualisation – to help support calmness – see page 159.
- Self-awareness with body outlines – *How do I feel now?* The client can compare any previous body outline drawings that might indicate a "before" and "after" or "then" and "now" state.

Stage 5: The Way Forward

Support for Planning, Problem-Solving, Strategy Formulation and Creativity

Stage 5 supports client creativity in their formulation of life strategies and new directions. It may include some time with problem-solving. In Stage 5 the client is assisted to plan ways to regulate affect outside of the counselling room; to stabilise impulsivity; and to recall resilience and strengths identified in session. It can include the formulation of behavioural plans that reinforce alternatives to acting-out, and can lead to the identification of, and satisfaction of needs.

- Encourage the client to formulate strategies and practical, doable steps to resolve problems if possible, or adjust to managing ongoing stress from their environment;
- Help identify and set up support in preparing for potential upcoming encounters that could generate challenges;
- Discuss positive, productive use of energy and identify alternatives to acting-out pent-up energy and emotions;
- Explore hopes and future projects, new directions, new interests;
- Allow time to discuss how the client can connect with or remember their resourcefulness and positive qualities;
- Encourage development of a personal metaphor, or select an image or miniature that will act as a reminder of their resourcefulness and plans in the days between sessions. This could be sketched, photographed or simply memorised and called on to remind the client of their new directions, strengths, plans and interests.

Optional Homework and Self-Care

This is an optional stage; the intention is to reinforce gains made in the client's wellbeing and practice ways to effectively self-manage and self-care. Although it can be quite empowering, this optional stage need not be offered in every session. Home-play might be a better, if not so easy, term! The task for the therapist is to monitor their own concepts of this stage; homework and self-care strategies are not designed to become a burden or demand on the client. Any achievement or non-achievement of the strategies can generate openness for guilt-free discussion.

Some inclusions as homework or self-care activities would be:

- Invite the client to make suggestions about what might remind them of therapeutic gains, their resilience and resourcefulness;
- Fun activities that facilitate and confirm a positive self-image;
- Activities to moderate excess energy, e.g., trampoline, walks, bicycle rides, etc.;
- For adolescent clients: Reflection with journal writing – see page 104;
- Communication "games" with parents or carers – where the setting supports this.

This ET 5-Stage Model offers a structure that can be used in both planning and clinical notes to record engagement in activities and outcomes observed during a session. A simple pro forma can be constructed listing the five or six stages and used to capture data relevant to the work done, as well as therapist reflections on what might be most useful in future sessions.

Building Rapport and Therapeutic Relating

Why Is Therapeutic Alliance Important?

This book shares over 70 therapeutic activities suitable for the support of young clients. We have found these activities to be most engaging for young clients, to assist them in investing time and energy into the therapeutic process. The focus in this section is on recommendations for building an effective client/therapist relationship, which can increase their motivation to participate.

Very early in Western psychotherapy Freud (1958), Rogers (1951) and Zetzel (1956) made claims that a positive connection with clients was a basic requirement for effective treatment. While there is some disagreement about the exact components of alliances, there is broad agreement that the relationship in counselling is crucial (Lambert & Ogles, 2004). The psychotherapy and counselling literature identifies the therapeutic alliance as one of the reliable ways to predict positive outcome (Luborsky & Luborsky, 2006).

Research into what promotes positive therapy outcomes makes it clear that growth and change are related to what clients engage with in sessions, what theories underlie the methods we use, but is most strongly influenced by how we relate to clients as individuals, and our ability to engage them in the process. Good techniques are associated with a good alliance (Muran & Barber, 2010), however, the manner in which interventions are applied can influence the alliance, i.e., both over-structuring and under-structuring therapy predict a negative alliance.

In attempting to develop an alliance with a young client, we should move back and forth between initiating and responding (Baylis et al., 2011), between *doing* and *being*, *leading* and *following*. Baylis et al. (2011) identified further behaviours on which alliance – according to their young clients – was dependent: Being nice, active listening and expressions of caring.

Counsellors need to pay particular attention to the relationship with the client and find ways to enhance what the client contributes to therapy. As ET is activity based, it can readily engage young clients who often prefer to "do something" rather than talk about difficult events or feelings. If you are an experienced counsellor, none of this is likely to appear to be new information. However, we like to emphasise the importance of taking time to develop a connection prior to offering ET activities, or indeed any intervention.

Relational Aims of Expressive Therapists

An ET approach to counselling involves three foundational components:

- how to *be* – the counsellor's mindfulness practice of developing therapeutic presence;
- how to *connect* – developing the relationship with the client;
- what to *do* – the activities that can be catalysts for communication and can engage a client.

In summary, the concepts that inform the ET relational style include development of a counsellor's capacity to remain curious and present; counsellor self-awareness; as well as their ability to feel and convey acceptance and compassion; professional skill with an invitational relating style; openness to intuitive guidance (Stickle & Arnd-Caddigan, 2019), and willingness to flow with creativity in spontaneous responding.

Counsellor Personal Development

Counsellor ways of being and relating depend to a large extent on their personal development. Therapist personal development can be seen as a career-long commitment to engage in collaborative reflection on both life experience and practice, and this can lead to new ways of understanding therapy and clients, as well as learning new ways of being with others (McLeod & McLeod, 2014). Personal development is a well-established core in Person-centred Therapy training; however, it is not a requirement in many approaches.

In personal development, what is it that has to be developed? It will be valuable for therapists to gain abilities with psychological flexibility, fluidity in moving between activity-based relating to intersubjective connection, discernment of client states and their openness and readiness for empathy or challenge. Personal development will enable comfort with the dance of following a client's lead or sometimes "leading" a client in order to support their self-discovery.

The key aspects of this development include a willingness to operate from a field of openness and professional curiosity about a client's psyche; discovering how a young person best processes information and expresses themselves. In addition, careful observation of the client requires consideration of what is taking place in the session without the need for immediate answers. Curiosity, openness and careful observation of the client's emotional, psychological and somatic states might lead to a raft of questions in the therapist's mind, and working from this state of questioning will contribute to openness.

Simple as it may sound, meeting a client "where they are", "joining with" them in whatever mood or state they may present in, can support a feeling of safety for them and may be a prerequisite for rapport. Can we work through any need for the client to fit, or validate, our framework? For example, an expressive therapist, with their vast array of experiential activities, needs to be equally comfortable supporting clients who are highly verbal, prefer to be logical/mathematical, show little interest in crayons and paper or miniatures, and want to focus on problem-solving.

Clients' self-reflection will be possible once feelings of safety can be tested and start to consolidate. If they feel safe enough to relax resistance or experiential avoidance, the next step involves a willingness to encounter their internal world. To help a client connect with emotion, follow their thoughts, deepen their somatic awareness and identify their wants and needs requires a counsellor to begin to understand what might be appropriate for them, as well as what might be problematic. Facing similar steps in our personal development will provide an ideal background to pursuing flexible and compassionate relating. In one of his earlier works, Rogers (1951) points out that our own personal development may determine our ability to be person-centred.

Trust

In an ET session, the therapeutic relationship begins by developing inner and outer trust. Outer trust grows through meeting the counsellor, feeling their acceptance and through a simple and clear framework for the processes. Inner trust, trust in self, develops through self-exploration that reveals both strengths and challenges. Young clients can learn to share their hunches, motivations and deepest fears when trust develops.

How do we *be* and relate in a way that will develop trust and safety? Research from neuroscience and psychotherapy over many years provides supportive evidence that a counsellor needs, ideally, to be in a regulated and present state to allow clients to risk dropping experiential avoidance and exploring their emotions and understanding and changing their behaviours. For example, consider Porges' (1995) polyvagal theory related to clients' nervous systems detecting safety; Geller and Greenberg's (2012) therapeutic present experiment; Dunn, Callahan, Swift and Ivanovic's (2013) positive impact of pre-session centring.

Internal trust refers to a client's capacity to see themselves as successful clients and with the ET activities. For example, an adolescent client who has never before used miniatures as symbols to explore an issue of loss or grief might at first wonder how their distress could be eased simply by picking some small objects off a shelf and arranging them on a table. Gradually, they come to see that these spontaneous actions begin to open windows to their thoughts, feelings and needs, and start to trust spontaneity within therapy. Is there a way our relating with a client can enhance their openness to vulnerability and self-awareness? When they feel safe, we can offer questions or activities that direct their awareness within.

What to Do?

Whenever possible, offer self-awareness, self-reflection and self-expression opportunities. These may be times of quiet sharing using drawing or choosing miniatures, or might involve accessing and expressing strong emotion through emotion-focused processes (see Chapter 7). Ideally, we want to relate to clients in a way that assists them to re-establish connection with their resourcefulness and self-efficacy. A therapeutic alliance that assumes clients have the capacities and internal resources to solve their problems, even if these seem distant or unknowable when first entering therapy, can support this re-connection.

After emotional challenges begin to ease, and a client feels support for growth in their sense of self, they can more readily reconnect with their personal resources and creative potential. Positive choices are then more likely, and clients are more likely to become productive and formulate positive action steps.

In the later stages of an ET session (see 5-Stage Model, p. 36), stimulate the client's formulation of their own strategies, action steps and ways of gaining support to achieve their aims. While restraint is practised from making overt suggestions, appropriateness of strategies a client can conceive is discussed in detail and feedback is given by the counsellor as to their suitability in relation to overall goals.

Invitations Rather than Instructions

A deeply person-centred – and therefore empowering – way of professional relating centres around offering invitations. An invitation calls for a response, a reflection, a choice; and with that, increased motivation to participate. If we hear ourselves saying; *I am interested in ...; I want you to ...; Could you ...?* these are rephrased as *Would you be willing to ...? Would you like to tell me about ...? See if you would like to ...* Invitations also bring opportunities for clients' boundaries to be acknowledged and respected in cases where they are not ready to respond to invitations. Invitations encourage the client to reflect on their needs, choices and increase their commitment and motivation to participate in the session (Baloche, 1996).

There is often a perception in novice therapists that efforts to establish empathy mean they need to use clever questioning and multiple guesses about what a client is feeling or thinking. This means that what sounds like a question can sometimes mask a statement. Could we say *"I wonder if you'd be able to share what's happening for you right now?"* rather than *"It sounds like you may be stuck/sad/angry/lost, etc."* The task is to take a step back from being the director of the process, while at the same time guiding the conversation, providing options, offering choices.

Encouraging a client to connect internally and discern their motivations, their wants and wishes and worries, means allowing time during the session for them to reflect, time for them to "hear" what they have discovered. Hence, the process of therapy moves to a holding space of "allowing", rather than a space of continual "doing". We would not want our young clients to merely be submissive responders in relation to our directions. We would want them to know that within therapy they are able to query, retain privacy, enact some control and have their preferences respected. This means asking something like *"When you tune in to your body and feelings, could you see what needs to happen next?"* This is more respectful than guessing what is happening and giving an instruction, or telling them to do something.

Examples of invitational relating or questioning:

- *Is there a way you would like to begin our time together today? For example, is there something you want to talk about? Would you like to share what is happening through drawing, writing, or choosing miniatures?*
- *Would you be willing to say more about that?*
- *Do you feel ready to move on?*
- *Would you be able to say something about what you are feeling?*
- *Would you be willing to share your drawing/worksheet/symbol work picture?*

There Are Many Ways to Build Rapport

Not surprisingly, Stage 1 of our 5-Stage Model for an ET session (see more on this on page 36) focuses on building rapport, a first step in building a strong therapeutic alliance. This first stage aims to "break the ice", clear the way, build rapport and allow the counsellor to learn about the client. Some have found rapport can develop very quickly, even within the first ten minutes of the first session, and it can strengthen over time. Counsellors in schools reported that working with ET greatly assisted rapport development (Pearson, 2003).

The counsellor's most usual contribution to developing rapport is the provision of active listening, meeting the client, encouraging, hearing and accepting their story. This can happen during a seemingly casual conversation, as well as through a more structured activity. To build client trust in this early stage we also need to provide opportunities for the client's apprehension, resistance or anxiety to be addressed, brought into the open, accepted and normalised.

An essential component of trust and rapport-building is providing some framework or rationale for counselling and for the myriad of activities that can be offered. We have found that many young clients have vague – or no – notions of what counselling is and what will be "expected" of them. Finding a simple way to communicate this is highly likely to reduce their apprehension and support a more truthful exchange. Within this framework, of course, is explaining confidentiality and its limitations.

There are many basic counselling skills that contribute to developing rapport; for example, allowing silence, giving the young client time to think and feel before launching forward with more questions. Many ET activities provide a framework for clients to reflect, to "gather their thoughts" and connect with their internal experience prior to sharing their stories. Reflecting back and paraphrasing, when used occasionally, can contribute here. As Rogers discovered, helping the client experience empathy may be one of the main ways to strengthen rapport.

Developing Rapport – Advice to Interns and New Counsellors

Stay open to what might be needed:

Remain fluid and flexible with therapeutic options, discuss these with clients, learn about and respect their preferences. Stay open to all ways of understanding (e.g., intellectual, emotional, somatic, etc.) what may be needed in each moment. Regularly seek feedback and support through clinical supervision.

Client as expert:

Begin with discovering what is most interesting to the client. Support the client's trust in their perceptions, even if they contain misunderstandings. Offer open, multiple-choice questions that are constructed as catalysts for recall, reflection and communication. Use your best efforts at analysis of the client's situation to guide and frame these questions, and offer them tentatively, knowing that our assumptions will often miss the mark. And, of course, stay open to remaining silent as they are, at times, drawn into playing with media, with little acknowledgement of our presence. Regard the client as the expert in themselves, even if they appear to be distant from their self-knowledge.

Trust the process:

Work from a perspective that a client cannot be wrong in what they focus on or what they express, or when they are ready to communicate. While with experience, we might have valid ideas on what to focus on and how to proceed, we do not know the client's needs for protection of vulnerability, their need to develop trust slowly, need to defend against connection with memories or difficult emotions. We respect their need to defend, so we aim to develop safety so that there is no need to protect.

When trust is established:

When clients feel safe, accessing and resolving difficult background or implicit experiences is supported through multiple means. For example, through emotion-focused processes that involve creating imaginary encounters and exploration through symbolic expression. Symbolic expression provides a safe outlet, that may incorporate imagination, metaphor, the use of miniatures, or process art. Symbolic expression provides opportunities for somatic and emotional release and can clear the way for understanding behaviour and sources of beliefs about self.

ACTIVITIES THAT BUILD RAPPORT

Activity 2.1 First Session Rapport Activity: *Pictures in Stone*

Materials: Collection of interesting stones (different shapes, textures, colours, markings on them) in an attractive bowl, candle in secure candle holder, large matches or lighter.

Aim: A time of focused attention that invites reflection and begins self-exploration.

Note: Please consider context, safety and client's emotional state. It may be appropriate, and risk-conscious, to forgo actual candle lighting.

1. Client is invited to light a small candle as a short opening – and later closing – ritual.
2. Client is invited to browse the stones and choose one they particularly like or that seems most interesting to them. Counsellor may select one as well.
3. Suggest the client hold the stone for a moment. Invite the client to take a couple of slow breaths, relax their body as much as possible, feel the stone's temperature, size, weight and texture.
4. Invite them to then look carefully at the stone, and see if there are any pictures or stories that this stone might evoke.

   - They are asked whether the markings might remind them of anything.
   - Invite the client to talk about whether the stone would have a mood.
   - Invite the client to describe the "picture" they see or the "story" that goes with their stone.

   The conversation does not need to have a direction or specific outcome. The aim is to help the client settle, while inviting them to engage, to connect on a level which is not directly and immediately related to the presenting problem.

   The counsellor may:

   - inquire if the picture or story relates to their life in any way, or reminds them of anything
   - simply encourage any conversation with gentle questioning
   - offer an activity next that relates to the emerging conversation.

   Client may like to keep the stone beside them during their session, then return it to the bowl at the end.

5. At the end of the session, the client is invited to extinguish the candle.

Activity 2.2 Role Play for Deepening Rapport: *My Favourite Toy*

Materials: Client brings to the session, or is asked to recall a favourite toy, and/or sketches it.

Aim: To provide a link between the therapy room and home life, to invite into the session something familiar and comforting, and to provide an opportunity for new clients to express hesitations about attending the session.

The client shows their toy, or draws it. Short general discussion inviting the client to tell you about their favourite toy. The counsellor then invites the client to role-play the toy.

- The client is encouraged to take some deep breaths between questions and to relax and bring awareness to their sensations and feelings.
- The client is encouraged to role-play the toy, responding to the following questions, in role as the toy, beginning each time: *"I …"* if possible.

- Counsellor says: *Could you take two big breaths and pretend you are this toy? Even if it seems a bit strange, could you:*
  - *Imagine you are changing now into the toy? Imagine you even look like the toy.*
  - *See if you can close your eyes for a moment if it helps to concentrate on your toy.*
  - *Do you want to change the way you are sitting, or stand, or take the shape of the toy?*
  - *See if you can imagine you are this toy now!*
  - *I am going to ask the toy a few questions. Let's see how the toy would answer.*

1. *Could you describe yourself as this toy? Can you tell me what you look like, your colours? Shapes? Your size?*
2. *Could you tell me what is inside you? And how do you feel about what is inside you?*
3. *What are you for? Who uses you, and why?*
4. *Do you make any sounds or movements? Could you show these now or tell me about the sounds or movements?*
5. *Do you, toy, have any special message for* …… (client's name), *or anything you would like to say to them? Any comment, any advice?*
6. *Now that* …… (client name) *is able to listen to you, is there anything else you would like to say?*

Pause

Could you take another full breath and finish being the toy? Come back to being a person. Take a moment to look around you. Take in the colours and shapes of the room. Now you are yourself again. Can you say something about how you feel now? How do you feel about the message from the toy?

Integration

- Invite the client to write down the message and any thoughts they have about that message (For a young client, write it down for them).
- Invite the client to talk about how they feel about the message, and if it could help them in their life.
- Discuss any links between the message and the client's daily life.

Note: For clients over 11–12 years, consider changing "toy" to "favourite activity or favourite thing you like to play with" – something that helps them relax and "chill out".

Parents and Carers: Building Connections with Supportive Others

This section is intended primarily for novice or intern counsellors. It offers some practical guidelines for engaging parents and carers to support their child's or adolescent's therapeutic process. Parental behaviour prior to, during and immediately after the first session can make a positive or negative impact on clients' willingness to participate and return to counselling.

Before First Session

During the pre-session phone or in-person intake interview, maintain the purpose of the interview: to gather some preliminary information and respond to questions the parent may have about counselling. In our early days, there were some times when a pre-session intake interview could move quickly towards becoming a pseudo-counselling session for the parent. This was understandable, as many parents and carers have often not considered seeking support for themselves. Another challenge was that, as a therapist in private practice, answering the phone meant the caller had direct access to a trained "listener". This meant the conversation could divert easily to parental distress, becoming less about the person for whom help was being sought.

In an intake interview aim to clarify the main reason for requesting counselling for the young person. Seek clarification about significant issues such as:

- attachment or trauma history
- client health history, physical issues or challenges, medications
- siblings: age gaps, relationships with siblings, any health issues for siblings
- family structure, family environment and any changes in family relationships
- school environment and client attitudes towards school
- social networks
- any recent changes or moves to a new location.

The client's attachment to family pets and any recent changes with family pets may be relevant. Typical intake information will also include the client's age, hobbies/interests, information about medications as well as time of taking medications. If an afternoon session is booked, recommend the client has a snack before the session. Engagement and focus can be diminished if blood sugar levels drop significantly.

We encourage counsellors not to assume parents or carers – or even the client – may know about or understand the causes of changes in the behaviour of their young ones. If there are any verbal or written reports from teachers or school staff, these may provide insight for a preliminary conceptualisation of the case. However, caution is needed not to create or solidify assumptions that could bias our therapeutic interactions.

For instance, MP had a 12-year-old male client whose family had moved from the suburbs to acreage just beyond the town perimeter, about two years prior to the session. The boy's parents had become concerned about their son's wellbeing because he was not thriving at his new, smaller school. He appeared to be disinterested in making new friends. Teachers and parents worried about this serious lack of interest in socialising and wondered if there might be some social dysfunction.

When simply asked about this at his first session, he was clear that he avoided making friends, as this would constitute being unfaithful to his old friends. In the family's excitement about the move to acreage, they neglected to support their children in farewelling friends and grieving separations. The session allowed the client to recall the "old days", creating pictures of past positive interactions, and to grieve this separation with tears. After this session he requested his parents set up a get-together with his old friends. After two sessions he had commenced social interactions and presented with enhanced wellbeing.

Enquire of parents and carers if they have read your website or read the brochure about your service. It is helpful to know how much they understand about the counselling process, what expectations they have, any personal history they may have with counselling, and what may be realistic outcomes. In particular, expressive therapists may need to briefly explain playful ways of working with arts-based tools. Should a young client claim they spent the session "playing", this is then unlikely to alarm parents or agency managers paying for the service. A simple explanation can be given that ET includes a range of modalities, offered from a client-centred attitude, within a paradigm of developing empowerment, that leads to enhanced outcomes.

If possible, find out whether the child or adolescent has agreed to attend counselling, whether they have asked for more emotional support from outside the family system, or whether they are resistant to the concept of speaking with a counsellor. Invite the parent or carer to reflect on how they will inform the child or adolescent about the appointment, and how they might explain counselling to a child who has not asked to "talk with someone". Many parents are unclear how to explain what counselling is and their reasons for wanting their child to access this type of support. Although, happily, this is less likely compared to 30 years ago when we first opened our practices.

> *Some years ago, HW worked with a 12-year-old boy whose father set up an appointment for what was referred to by the parent as a much-needed "emergency" counselling session. On the day, the nominated client was puzzled why he was in my office. When Dad was invited into the session and asked about the call for an "emergency" session, the parent said that when he was 12 years old he had no one to talk with about things that were bothering him. He wanted his son to be able to talk freely about his feelings.*

Back in 1998, a graduate of our course devised a 'letter' to parents of her young clients. The letter was straightforward and simple, with the aim of helping parents and carers understand the difference between their perceptions and expectations of therapy, and the realities of conducting therapy with a young person. Very generously, she gave the authors permission to share her letter. Almost three decades since this was created, the letter has proved extremely useful in easing the concerns parents may have about why ET would be a way to help their child or adolescent. These are her words:

> **Letter to Parents and Carers: About Counselling with Expressive Therapies**
>
> *Some of the techniques used in counselling children are a little different from those used with adults.*
>
> *Your child may tell you that they played a game, drew a picture, played with toys or played in a sandbox. You may think this is a very odd way to get to the bottom of whatever the problem is, or you may think it doesn't sound very helpful in developing "healthier" strategies in life.*
>
> *However, as you would understand, if I were simply to invite a child to talk to me, they would probably feel hesitant and uncomfortable about telling me their concerns. This is why I combine verbal counselling with other strategies, such as the use of games, art media or work with symbols and sand. These strategies are intended to help children feel more at ease and provide them with alternative or additional means of communication.*
>
> *If given the opportunity, children are able to tell their story, sort out a problem or gain a sense of control over an issue. My role is to facilitate this process, and sometimes, I cannot explain precisely what has helped the child feel better.*

I believe the most helpful things you, as parents, can do are:

- *Provide opportunities for your child to talk about the work they are doing with me, if they wish to.*
- *Do not continue to question them if they seem unwilling to talk about it now.*
- *Be accepting when your child expresses strong feelings.*
- *Provide the usual limits on unacceptable or destructive behaviour.*
- *Remember that you know your child better than anyone else, including me, so please share your opinions and observations.*
- *Do not hesitate to telephone me if you want to discuss anything between sessions.*

At the First Session

At the first session, familiarise the client and parent with the consulting room, waiting area, and bathroom facilities. Discuss the client's choice of having the parent in the room or nearby. If the client wants a parent to be with them, arrange a signal to the parent for when you think it may be appropriate for them to leave. This would, of course, be done in consultation with the young client. Having a parent beside them can initially be supportive; however, if rapport develops well with the counsellor, having the parent in the room may become limiting.

Parents and carers are often interested in how long the therapeutic process might take. It is useful to explain that counselling is a process over time, and it is not possible to be exact. Invite feedback from parents' evaluations and observations after their child or adolescent has completed a number of sessions. Clarify that your role as a counsellor is not to offer a diagnosis or explanations for issues that lead to parents seeking counselling for their child. It can be ideal to request initial attendance for at least three sessions, after which time a parent can assess effectiveness or suitability. Some therapists have noted positive changes may be evident after about 6 to 8 sessions for young clients (e.g., Kalff, 2003) and research indicates 8 to 10 sessions with adults (Lambert et al., 1994); and this can be a useful guide to give primary caregivers/parents. However, it is not unusual for some changes in mood, behaviour, and optimism to be evident after the first session.

Clarity on the administration of sessions is essential; such as the duration of sessions: Recommend 45 to 60 minutes for children (depending on age and interest levels), and perhaps 75 minutes for adolescents. The typical frequency of sessions should be discussed, with a suggestion that sessions be weekly at first, or if the issue is urgent and impacting, a few days apart to begin with. Perhaps after 6 to 8 weeks, if symptoms are decreasing, move to fortnightly appointments. For adolescents, incrementally expand the time between sessions around the time of the eighth session. Remember to make sure parents and carers have clarity about the cost of service, and the method and timing of payments. However, if clients are in recovery from trauma, and Stage 1 of our model remains a central focus, it is helpful to plan for some long-term support.

Confidentiality for young clients must be ensured as much as possible. The child is the client, and they have the usual rights to confidentiality. Obviously, the limits of confidentiality must also be made very clear. Clarify that parents would not normally be in the consulting room during ET sessions. However, a young client can be invited to choose if they want a parent with them initially. Counsellors should always aim to discuss with a young client a need to expand confidentiality to parents and carers.

At completion of the first session, before the client leaves the consulting room, support them to reflect on what they might want to share about the session with others and what session artefacts might go home or remain in the consulting room. There are times when it will be appropriate to revisit the boundaries of confidentiality at the end of a session.

Naturally, parents and carers want and seek feedback on the therapeutic process. It can be helpful to indicate any possible behavioural outcomes from the session, possible adjustment symptoms, moods, emotional needs in the 24–48 hour period immediately following the session. Young clients need to be informed that the therapist will, more often than not, have a brief discussion with the parent/carer to keep that person informed about the direction of therapy. The client needs confirmation that the content of the session will not be shared without express permission from the client (with the usual ethical exceptions).

If possible, make an appointment time for a parent/carer to make contact to discuss the first session. No details of what the child discussed are revealed during this discussion. What is available for discussion with a parent is information about the therapeutic relationship and their young person's engagement within the session. After the session, some very broad general and perhaps supportive comments about how the session went can be shared in the presence of the client. Make it clear to the parent/carer that feedback will not be provided immediately after the session, and definitely not in the presence of the young person. The client needs to be able to leave the session with their dignity intact, and with their emerging sense of rapport and trust with the therapist. Furthermore, they may still be processing their experiences in the session; therefore, premature commentary is unlikely to be helpful.

In preparing to discuss the case with parents or carers, reflect on ways it may be possible to harness their interest to help the child. When providing feedback, report a positive aspect of the session. Consider if you can normalise the problem, for example: Is the client's behaviour developmentally normal? Invite them to give you feedback, request their observations about any changes and emotional state after the session, e.g.: *"How was Tim on the way home?" "How was Jenny over the next few days or over the week?"* Point out any changes they notice in relation to the frequency and seriousness of presenting problem(s), as some parents may unknowingly "shift the goal posts".

Important to the child's progress in therapy is establishing who provides emotional support to parents/carers. This can be a delicate topic for discussion and may not be considered relevant by them. However, parents' states of wellbeing can have a significant impact on therapeutic outcomes. Is there a way to inquire if they have a support network? Is it appropriate to consider if there might be value in, or the possibility of, them seeking counselling support or participation in family therapy?

Post-Session Discussions and Home Support

Part of a post-session discussion with parents or carers may include suggestions for supporting integration of the session at home. If there is a willingness and openness to this, offer one or two ideas on how parents or carers can support the client at home. These might include:

- Provide clear signals to your child that you are interested in listening.
- Provide 100% focus on your child when listening to their communication.
- Arrange some individual one-on-one time with your child.
- Increase activities that involve physical expression and movement (as opposed to passive entertainment).
- Offer some foot or hand massage, some form of positive touch that may be shared.
- Set up a creative/drawing space to encourage regular expression and sharing of feelings together with their child.
- Create or colour in mandalas, or simply doodle. When a parent can participate in creative activities, a child can benefit from feeling accompanied and from spontaneous sharing of concerns.
- Review and decrease passive time with screens, reduce exposure to TV, video games and hypnotic YouTube distractions. Always offer expressive alternatives.
- Follow negative instruction with a positively geared comment – follow "don't" with "do" or "not that, but try this".
- Find ways of relating to their child that enhance self-esteem, e.g., ask their opinion more often, give encouragement, use "I" messages, involve client in problem-solving.
- Allow some unstructured alone time. Initially, this may not be popular; nevertheless, developmentally, time alone can be an important experience for them, particularly in the digital age where there can be a tendency to fill all space and time with incoming stimuli.
- Lastly, provide a positive model – "Think well of yourself" (Oaklander, 1978).

As you get to know a client, consider if further referral might be recommended. Might the child or family benefit from additional support? For example, is there evidence of benefit from educational testing, extra educational support, or psychological testing? Might the family benefit from social work support and/or family therapy? What are the pragmatics of the situation? What is possible now? What can be delayed until a later stage? What part can you play in supporting the growth and wellbeing of the young person, in relation to the context of family?

Adapting ET Activities

ET activity formats are somewhat like recipes. Once you are familiar with the principles of cooking and the approximate ratios of ingredients, you can vary some of the ingredients and create with different emphasis. In adapting our "recipes", the structured activities, apply your creativity to match the client(s)' needs or interests. Consider a client's readiness to engage; cognitive, language, motor and emotional skills level; cultural background (social, familial, belief systems); vocabulary range; interests and hobbies; and preferred intelligences. The main principle is to collaborate with your client to structure a session and adapt activities to accommodate client preferences.

Setting the Scene – Getting Started

This checklist assumes completion of a core level of experiential ET, prior to applying this therapeutic approach.

Before a Client Arrives

Review each potential activity you may be planning to offer. Consider if the language is appropriate for the age of the client or their cultural background. Always explore the activities yourself prior to offering to a client. This supports an ability to assess the suitability of the activity for a particular client, as well as your confidence in presenting and/or adapting the activity.

Review case notes. Take some time to be curious about your client, their preferred way of working in therapy (if known or able to be assessed), and their emotional needs. It could be that their experience of our genuine curiosity can catalyse self-reflection. If you plan to incorporate recorded music as a focal activity or as background, familiarise yourself with sound equipment before the client arrives, check music suitability, decide on specific tracks and have options for music tracks to support specific emotions.

For a new client, review the suggestions for Stages 1 and 2 of the 5-Stage Model (see page 36). Plan several rapport-building discussion topics and activities.

When the Client Arrives

Take time to find out as much as you can about who they are, without becoming an inquisitor. You could discuss:

- their aims for counselling in general – if they have any (even if you know parents' aims). Acknowledge that as a "mandated" client they may not have thought about this;
- their understanding of counselling and its purpose;
- how you work and provide a rationale for counselling and your style;
- the conditions for confidentiality;
- the safety required for taking home any drawings, photographs or writing.

After meeting the client and providing some orientation to your consulting room and available materials, offer choices in activities. For each activity, offer a brief overview of the aim and rationale before presenting.

Find out from your client if they feel willing to participate; what will "work" for them.

Think of yourself as a companion, sit to the side of the client, in a seating arrangement that is non-confrontational.

If there appears to be hesitancy or resistance in the client towards the session, or to a particular activity, encourage them to talk about their concerns or what is not working, what might work better, what they prefer. Respectfully bring their hesitation into the open. Find out if they would prefer to focus on something else or prefer you to offer something different.

As the session progresses, consider and reflect on any possible transference and counter-transference issues, for example if the client responds to you as an authority figure. This is for your information. While ET does not focus on working through the transference directly, it provides multiple ways transference can be expressed or acknowledged through projection onto art creations, symbol arrangements, or written artefacts, etc. Working in a person-centred way, being genuine, is most likely to help them relate more directly to you.

References

Ahuja, S., & Saha, A. (2016). They lead, you follow: Role of non-directive play therapy in building resilience. *Journal of Psychosocial Research*, *11*(1), 167–175.

Austin, S. F. (1917). *Principles of drama-therapy* (Vol. 769, Harvard medicine preservation microfilm project). Sopherim.

Axline, V. M. (1947). *Play therapy: The inner dynamics of childhood*. Houghton Mifflin.

Axline, V. M. (1989). *Play therapy*. Churchill Livingstone.

Baloche, L. (1996). Clues about motivation and creativity. *Cooperative Learning*, *16*(3), 13–16.

Baylis, P. J., Collins, D., & Coleman, H. (2011). Child alliance process theory: A qualitative study of a child centred therapeutic alliance. *Child and Adolescent Social Work Journal*, *28*(2), 79–95.

Biley, F. C. (1999). Music as therapy: A brief history. *Complementary Therapies in Nursing and Midwifery*, *5*(5), 140–143.

Booth, P. B., & Jernberg, A. M. (2009). *Theraplay: Helping parents and children build better relationships through attachment-based play*. John Wiley & Sons.

Bosmans, G. (2016). Cognitive behaviour therapy for children and adolescents: Can attachment theory contribute to its efficacy? *Clinical Child and Family Psychology Review*, *19*(4), 310–328.

Bretherton, I. (1999). Updating the 'internal working model' construct: Some reflections. *Attachment & Human Development*, *1*(3), 343–357.

Bussing, R., Mason, D. M., Bell, L., Porter, P., & Garvan, C. (2010). Adolescent outcomes of childhood attention-deficit/hyperactivity disorder in a diverse community sample. *Journal of the American Academy of Child & Adolescent Psychiatry*, *49*(6), 595–605.

Cappas, N. M., Andres-Hyman, R., & Davidson, L. (2005). What psychotherapists can begin to learn from neuroscience: Seven principles of a brain-based psychotherapy. *Psychotherapy: Theory, Research, Practice, Training*, *42*(3), 374–383.

Catania, A., & Harnad, S. E. (1988). *The selection of behavior: The operant behaviorism of BF Skinner: Comments and consequences*. Cambridge University Press.

Cooper, M. (2004). Towards a relationally-orientated approach to therapy: Empirical support and analysis. *British Journal of Guidance & Counselling*, *32*(4), 451–460.

Corning, J. L. (1912). The musical memory and its derangement (Amusia). *The Medical Record: A Weekly Journal of Medicine and Surgery*, *81*, 51–62.

De Shazer, S., & Berg, I. K. (1997). 'What works?' Remarks on research aspects of solution-focused brief therapy. *Journal of Family Therapy*, *19*(2), 121–124.

Dunn, R., Callahan, J. L., Swift, J. K., & Ivanovic, M. (2013). Effects of pre-session centering for therapists on session presence and effectiveness. *Psychotherapy Research*, *23*(1), 78–85.

Frankel, J. B. (1998). The play's the thing – How the essential processes of therapy are seen most clearly in child therapy. *Psychoanalytic Dialogues*, *8*(1), 149–182.

Freud, S. (1958). *On creativity and the unconscious*. Harper.

Gardner, H. (2006). *Multiple intelligences. New horizons*. Basic Books.

Gendlin, E. (1999). Implicit entry and focusing. *The Humanistic Psychologist*, *27*(1), 80–88.

Geller, S. M., & Greenberg, L. S. (2012). *Therapeutic presence: A mindful approach to effective therapy*. American Psychological Association.

Gidley, J. (2005). Giving hope back to our young people: Creating a new spiritual mythology for Western culture. *Journal of Futures Studies*, *9*(3), 17–30.

Greenberg, L. S. (2004). Emotion–focused therapy. *Clinical Psychology & Psychotherapy: An International Journal of Theory & Practice*, *11*(1), 3–16.

Grof, S., Grof, C., & Kornfield, J. (2010). *Holotropic breathwork: A new approach to self-exploration and therapy*. SUNY Press.

Haley, J. (1976). *Problem-solving therapy*. Jossey-Bass.

Hammack, P. L. (2003). The question of Cognitive Therapy in a postmodern world. *Ethical Human Sciences and Services*, *5*(3), 209–224.

Haynes, S. N., & O'Brien, W. H. (1990). Functional analysis in behavior therapy. *Clinical Psychology Review*, *10*(6), 649–668.

Hendricks, M. N. (2007). The role of experiencing in psychotherapy: Attending to the "bodily felt sense" of a problem makes any orientation more effective. *Journal of Contemporary Psychotherapy*, *37*(1), 41–46.

Hetherington, A. (1999). A psychodynamic perspective on early childhood trauma in an adult: A case study. *Psychodynamic Counselling, 5*(1), 73–85.
Holmes, J. (2014). *John Bowlby and attachment theory.* Routledge.
Jacobs, M. (1988). *Psychodynamic counselling in action.* Sage Publications.
Jaskoski, H. (1980). Poetry, poetics and the poetry therapist. *The Arts in Psychotherapy, 7*(4), 275–279.
Johnson, S. M. (2018). *Attachment theory in practice: Emotionally Focused Therapy (EFT) with individuals, couples, and families.* Guilford Publications.
Kalff, D. M. (2003). *Sandplay: A psychotherapeutic approach to the psyche.* Temenos Press.
Lambert, M. J., Bergin, A. E., & Garfield, S. L. (1994). The effectiveness of psychotherapy. *Encyclopedia of Psychotherapy, 1,* 709–714.
Lambert, M. J., & Ogles, B. M. (2004). The efficacy and effectiveness of psychotherapy. In *Bergin and Garfield's handbook of psychotherapy and behavior change, 5,* 139–193.
Lowen, A., & Lowen, L. (2012). *The vibrant way to health.* Simon and Schuster.
Lowenfeld, M. (1950). The nature and use of the Lowenfeld World Technique in work with children and adults. *The Journal of Psychology, 30*(2), 325–331.
Luborsky, L., & Luborsky, E. (2006). *Research and psychotherapy. The vital link.* Rowman & Littlefield Publishers.
McLeod, J., & McLeod, J. (2014). *Personal and professional development for counsellors, psychotherapists and mental health practitioners.* McGraw-Hill Education (UK).
Midgley, N., Hayes, J., & Cooper, M. (Eds.). (2017). *Essential research findings in child and adolescent counselling and psychotherapy.* Sage.
Minuchin, S. (1974). *Families and family therapy.* Harvard University Press.
Minuchin, S. (2014). The restoried history of family therapy. In J. K. Zeig (Ed.), *The evolution of psychotherapy: The second conference* (pp. 3–10). Routledge.
Moreno, J. D. (2014). *Impromptu man: JL Moreno and the origins of psychodrama, encounter culture, and the social network.* Bellevue Literary Press.
Muran, J. C., & Barber, J. P. (2010). *The therapeutic alliance. An evidence-based guide to practice.* The Guilford Press.
Naumburg, M. (1958). *Art therapy: Its scope and function in the clinical application of projective drawings.* Grune and Stratton.
Nichols, M. P., & Efran, J. S. (1985). Catharsis in psychotherapy: A new perspective. *Psychotherapy: Theory, Research, Practice, Training, 22*(1), 46–58.
Oaklander, V. (1978). *Windows to our children: A Gestalt therapy approach to children and adolescents.* Gestalt Journal.
Pearce, J. W., & Pezzot-Pearce, T. D. (1994). Attachment theory and its implications for psychotherapy with maltreated children. *Child Abuse & Neglect, 18*(5), 425–438.
Pearson, M. (2003). Guidance officer and counsellor perspectives on using expressive therapies to support students. *Australian Journal of Guidance and Counselling, 13*(2), 205–224.
Pearson, M., & Nolan, P. (2004). *Emotional release for children: Repairing the past, preparing the future.* Jessica Kingsley Publishers.
Pearson, M., & Wilson, H. (2009). *Using expressive arts to work with mind, body and emotions: Theory and practice.* Jessica Kingsley Publishers.
Perls, F. (1969). *Gestalt Therapy verbatim.* Gestalt Journal Press.
Porges, S. W. (1995). Orienting in a defensive world: Mammalian modifications of our evolutionary heritage. A polyvagal theory. *Psychophysiology, 32*(4), 301–318.
Porter, L. (2020). *Student behaviour: Theory and practice for teachers.* Routledge.

Rachman, S. (1993). A critique of cognitive therapy for anxiety disorders. *Journal of Behavior Therapy and Experimental Psychiatry*, *24*(4), 279–288.
Rachman, S. (2015). The evolution of behaviour therapy and cognitive behaviour therapy. *Behaviour Research and Therapy*, *64*, 1–8.
Reich, W. (1933/1980). *Character analysis*. Farrar, Straus and Giroux.
Rogers, C. R. (1951). *Client-centered therapy: Its current practice, implications, and theory*. Houghton Mifflin.
Rogers, C. R. (1961). *On becoming a person: A therapist's view of psychotherapy*. Houghton Mifflin.
Rothschild, B. (2000). *The body remembers: The psychophysiology of trauma and trauma treatment*. W.W. Norton & Company.
Samuels, A. (2003). *Jung and the post-Jungians*. Routledge.
Schore, A. N. (2000). Attachment and the regulation of the right brain. *Attachment & Human Development*, *2*(1), 23–47.
Schwarz, J. E. (2013). *Meaning and spirituality in adolescence: Practices and perspectives of school counselors*. Montclair State University.
Stickle, M., & Arnd-Caddigan, M. (2019). *Intuition in psychotherapy: From research to practice*. Routledge.
Vaughan, F. E. (2012). *The inward arc: Healing in psychotherapy and spirituality*. iUniverse.
Victoria, H. K., & Caldwell, C. (2013). Breathwork in body psychotherapy: Clinical applications. *Body, Movement and Dance in Psychotherapy*, *8*(4), 216–228.
Whitaker, C. A., & Keith, D. V. (1981). Symbolic-experiential family therapy. In A. S. Gurman & D. P. Kniskern (Eds.), *Handbook of family therapy* (Vol. 1, pp. 187–225). Routledge.
White, M. (2003). Narrative practice and community assignments. *International Journal of Narrative Therapy & Community Work*, *2*, 17–55.
Wiener, D. J., & Oxford, L. K. (2003). Introduction: Action methods in family therapy. In D. J. Wiener & L. K. Oxford (Eds.), *Action therapy with families and groups: Using creative arts improvisation in clinical practice* (pp. 15–17). American Psychological Association.
Zetzel, E. R. (1956). Current concepts of transference. *International Journal of Psychoanalysis*, *37*, 369–376.

3 Colour, Shape, Symbol and Image

Using Visual Media

Visual Media in Expressive Therapies

Exploring imagery – created, imagined or borrowed – as a core activity in ET has been shown to be effective in helping people change, as many writers have also observed over a long period of time (e.g., Lazarus, 1982; McNiff, 1992, 2004; Skovholt et al., 1989; Wolpe, 1958). Outcomes from skilful therapeutic help that includes accessing creative, expressive processes to activate self-healing in the psyche have the potential to lead to recovery from psychological distress (Eaton et al., 2007).

The formal discipline of Art Therapy is quite distinct from the ways visual art can be used in ET with child and adolescent clients. The term Art Therapist is one applied to a person who has specific training (usually at a post-graduate level) in that field. However, art and the use of colour, line, shape, image and miniatures has always been, and remains, an integral resource in the multimodal expressive therapies approach.

Like much of Western psychotherapy, art therapy emerged within the prevailing psychoanalytic paradigm early in the 20th century. The history of the use of art in therapy includes the work of Melanie Klein (1882–1960), who used art and toys with her young patients. Later, in the 1940s, Margaret Naumburg (1890–1983) named her approach ***dynamically oriented art therapy***. The core premise of her method was based on releasing the unconscious through spontaneous art expression (Coleman & Farris-Dufrene, 1996). Edith Kramer (1916–2014) practised Freudian ego psychology and concentrated on the therapeutic values in using art. Her goal for art therapy was: "leading toward personality growth and rehabilitation" (Kramer, 1958, p. 7). She explored the value of art in sublimation – a process wherein direct instinctive gratification is relinquished, and a substitute activity is found that permits symbolic gratification of the same need, in a socially productive way (Kramer, 1958).

Creating an image within therapy can enhance a client's willingness to communicate and can support a sense of becoming "unstuck", being able to "do something" (Oster & Montegomery, 1996). Creating and working with imagery can enhance a client's active involvement in the therapy process (Lusebrink, 1990; McNiff, 2004), and this engagement contributes to

DOI: 10.4324/9781003671879-3

positive outcomes. Using art as part of therapy provides access to a wider range of the multiple intelligences for learning, communication, and resolution. It allows expression of non-verbal thinking, provides an opportunity for pre-conscious and pre-verbal issues to emerge, and the creativity contributes to strengthening client resilience.

The inclusion in therapy of creative activities increases congruence for the client – building clearer connections between explicit awareness and implicit knowledge, as well as between emotion, cognition and somatic awareness. Creative expressive techniques engender action, activate new energy and provide reinforcement. Engaging with visual art can generate improved focus; enrich and expand self; establish a new sense of self; provide concreteness – evidence of progress with the personal journey; and development of insight (Gladding, 1998).

Psychological healing can be enhanced by accessing, symbolising and externalising internal conflicts so they can be recognised and worked with, through a range of expressive modalities (Malchiodi, 2005; McNiff, 2004). Creativity is also regarded as preventative as well as remedial (Gladding, 1998). From a Gestalt perspective, art was seen as an integrative process (Oaklander, 1988), making it ideal as part of the Five-Stage ET Model (see page 36).

There are a large number of research projects investigating art therapy (Boehm et al., 2014; Joschko et al., 2024; Payne, 1993). However, the wide range of variables within clients can make objective data gathering a challenge. In discussing the difficulties of research on the creative arts in counselling, researchers (e.g., Cohen-Yatziv & Regev, 2019; Gladding, 1998) have identified the difficulty of controlling and isolating variables that promote or hinder client growth. Kapitan (2011) points out the challenges in confirming a clear perspective from which to view art therapy outcomes. McNiff (2012) adds the refinement of identifying art therapy research that is arts-based, as compared with non-arts-based.

Art therapy has been shown to be valuable with clients affected by abuse and trauma, addictions, dementia, eating disorders, learning difficulties, offenders, those in palliative care; in the fields of depression, personality disorders, psychotic and related disorders; with children and adolescents affected by ADHD, Autistic Spectrum Disorders, and children affected by sexual abuse (Gilroy, 2006). According to Nabarro (2005), creating artwork can be a way for children to express traumatic experiences to their caregivers, providing them with a context within which to recognise, process and share their emotions (Berman, 2001).

Areas of benefit from using visual art methods include: Creating connection with the unconscious and identifying components of conflicts; symbolising feelings and helping externalise a distressing event; inspiring clients, engendering hope and helping clients contact the transcendent and growth side of their personality (Cohen-Yatziv & Regev, 2019; Gladding, 1998). Visual arts are non-threatening, self-interpreted and a medium that is extremely flexible and can easily be combined with other modes of expression.

Use of Imagery

Use of imagery has long been found to be an effective means to support a change process (Wolpe, 1958; Lazarus, 1982; Skovholt et al., 1989). Imagery enhances active involvement in the therapeutic process (Lusebrink, 1990), and strengthens the link between body, mind and emotion.

Within a pluralistic approach to counselling (Cooper & McLeod, 2011) there is an emphasis on respect for diversity. A pluralistic approach privileges clients' unique and individual ways they process and communicate information. Clients may have specific preferences about the direction and style of therapy. In a Cooper et al. (2023) study the recommendation is to open discussion on preferences early in therapy. Millard, et al. (2021) also found that clients' perceived capabilities were important factors in choosing a creative arts therapy.

We have encountered a few clients who report significant challenges to visualisation, otherwise known as aphantasia or *image-free thinking*. A person with aphantasia has difficulty creating a mental image, e.g., of familiar objects, people, or places or images of the future (Aphantasia Network). This means that, for participation in visualisations or activities where holding a mental image is central, it is ideal to have a set of miniatures that the client can select and arrange, rather than struggling to hold or develop an image in their mind.

Purposes of Visual Art in Expressive Therapies

There are four specific ways visual art is used in ET: (1) *Reflective Art* to support recall and assembling of concepts for therapeutic exploration; (2) *Self-awareness Art* to enhance emotional literacy, (3) *Process Art* to work through issues, as a venting or emotional release activity and (4) *Completion and Integration Art* to support closure of a process or a session.

Reflective Art: What's Been Happening around Me?

Reflective art is used to support recall and connection with memories, moods and emotions: E.g., remembering a sad or a happy time. The client is given time to recollect a time and place that is significant for them. They are invited to use art materials to give expression to, and consolidate that recollection. Expression using colours, lines and shapes may be representational and/ or abstract. Whatever form it takes, it will convey information, mood and reactions.

Sketching events such as holidays, family gatherings or emotionally charged moments generates reflection on the associated memories and can increase communication with the counsellor that can consolidate awareness and add to meaning making. Reflective art can include ways to reduce any negative self-belief about artistic expression, such as "I can't draw".

A natural phenomenon in the psyche, projection, the process through which disowned intra-psychic material can be externalised without immediate recognition of that process (Grant & Crawley, 2002). The projective mechanism comes alive in the creation of reflective art. There is what was intended by the art-maker, along with what emerges beyond their conscious intent. In reviewing their created image, the client may also project onto that image meanings and issues that unexpectedly appear relevant.

Projective techniques provide ideal intervention with clients whose life is characterised by a legacy of neglect, abuse and trauma. Projection allows them to be indirect in moving closer to difficult psychological material. Projective art activities can be ideal where a client experiences nervous system overload, or for whom re-traumatisation (even unwittingly), is to be avoided (Rothschild, 2000) (see Figure 3.1).

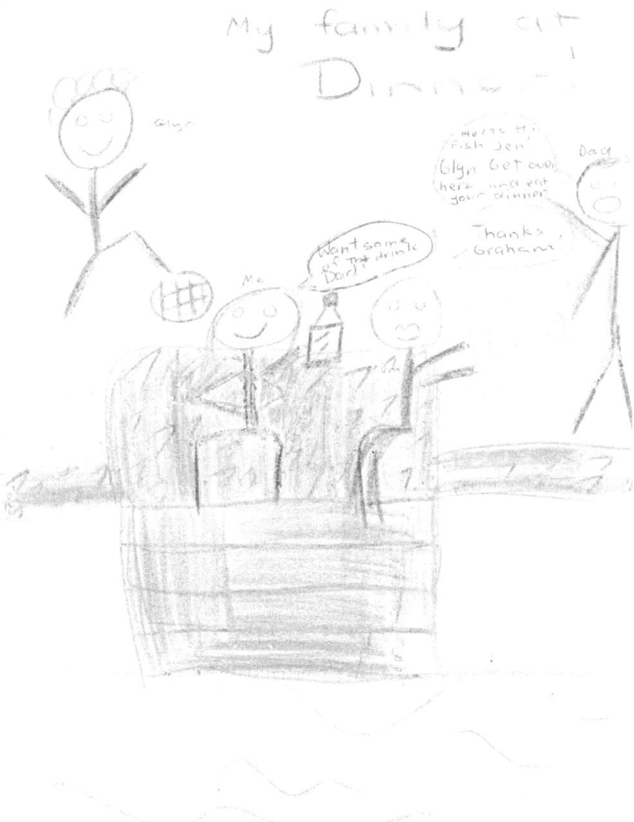
My family at
Glyn
Dad
Glyn Get over here and eat your dinner
Thanks Graham
Want some of that drink Dad?
Me

Figure 3.1 Reflective art – my family at dinner.

Mask-Making

Can contribute to both reflective and self-awareness art. Masks are an ancient means of changing identity and assuming a different persona. Designing masks enables clients to project their thoughts into objects that can be viewed as self-representative. With young clients, persona work involves exploring how they think they are seen by others and provides opportunities to momentarily be someone else. Masks have been used in individual and group settings to help clients of various ages explore: Identity and identity formation, to identify and integrate disowned emotions, to explore spirituality, to assume a different or more empowered self, and to find balance (Cavazos, 2012) (see Figure 3.2).

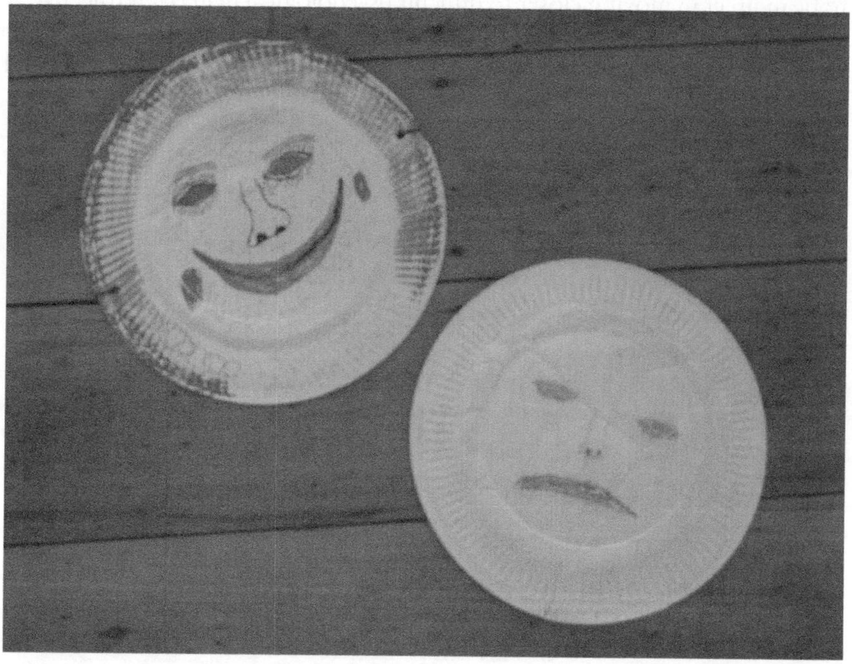

Figure 3.2 Reflective art – mask making.

Self-Awareness Art: What's Been Happening inside Me?

Self-awareness art includes the use of somatic focus and expression on body outlines as well as expressing feelings identified after self-awareness activities. A sketch created to show tensions is a form of emotional awareness art and can contribute to emotional literacy. A client is invited by the counsellor to take a minute or two (or more) to connect with self and to see if it is possible to locate the somatic aspect of a feeling (where in the body might the feeling be). The client is invited to then select colours and use shapes and lines to express the feeling. In some cases, it may be difficult to talk about feelings or to convey the strength, intensity, or emotion that accompanied an experience. Using colours, lines and shapes can be a means by which a client is able to express the inexpressible without needing to find language that the therapist will understand (see Figure 3.3).

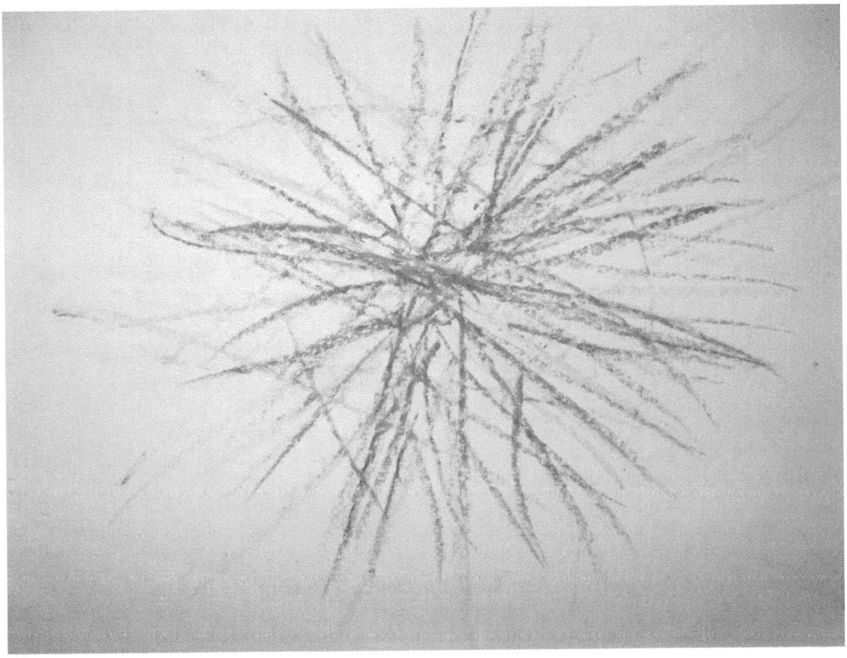

Figure 3.3 Self-awareness art – the feeling inside.

Process Art: Going with the Flow

To support access to and reflection on emotion, an invitation is offered to choose colours, lines, shapes, that best express a client's reactions to an event. The client begins to find ways to transfer internal experience onto a large sheet of paper. The client is gently encouraged to use the art materials (crayons, pencils, paints, etc.) continuously until the feeling or reaction is as fully expressed as possible. This could mean there are several pages of "drawing" created in rapid succession. Engaging in process art can be a valuable step in aiding the release of emotional and physical tension. These drawings are an in-the-moment process and usually are not retained after the session as they may no longer have significance for the client. Process art is, however, reviewed as a way for the client to track their experience of in-the-moment mood change. Process art can also be useful as "homework", as a self-support strategy for temporary relief from emotional stress. However, an ET therapist should be aware of and sensitive to safety issues and any implication/s for a young person for engaging in this process at home (see Figure 3.4).

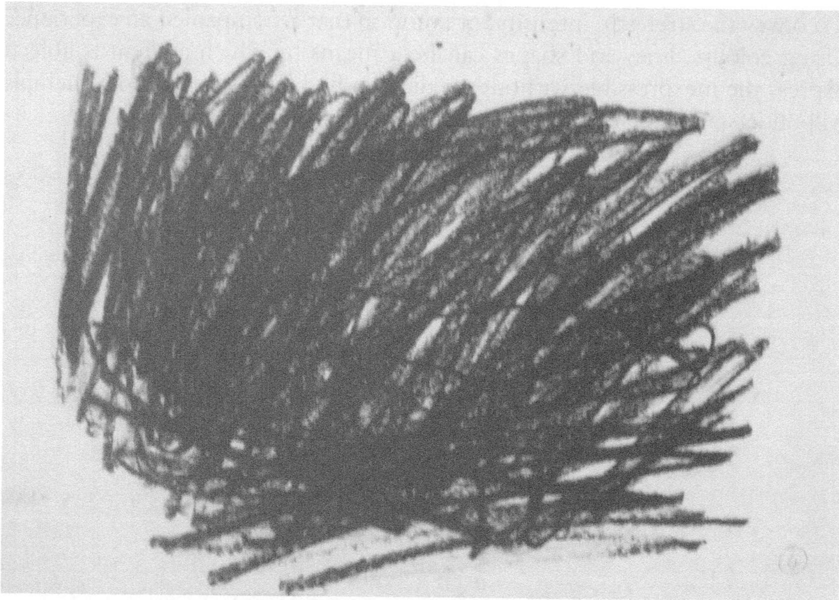

Figure 3.4 Process art – anger.

Completion and Integration Art: Cooling Down, Finding My Centre

The importance of the integration of a session is central to safe ET practice. Spending time with a completion drawing can allow the body to recover, mood to settle, understanding to emerge, and is essential after emotion-focused work. Completion art is usually produced as part of the fourth integration stage of a session and may be retained as a reminder of the experiences as well as for later review.

Body Outlines

Can be used by a client to express somatic and emotional awareness after completing an ET activity or a session. They can then compare their own state with internal experiences noted early in the session. In other words, as a way to identify changes and transformation.

Mandalas

Used as an integration option in ET. Drawing in a circle is a form of completion art. Mandala creation promotes a sense of control and concentration, and this focus can aid calmness and reflection at the end of a session. Using the circle as a framework, a client is invited to allow free expression in, around, over, or beyond the circle. A circle shape is one that suggests a centre and can bring a balancing, calming effect that evokes a sense of peacefulness. Mandala creation sometimes helps the client to focus, centre emotionally and cognitively into the task at hand while allowing the therapeutic components of the experience to assist emotional healing and integration (Fincher, 2009) (see Figure 3.5).

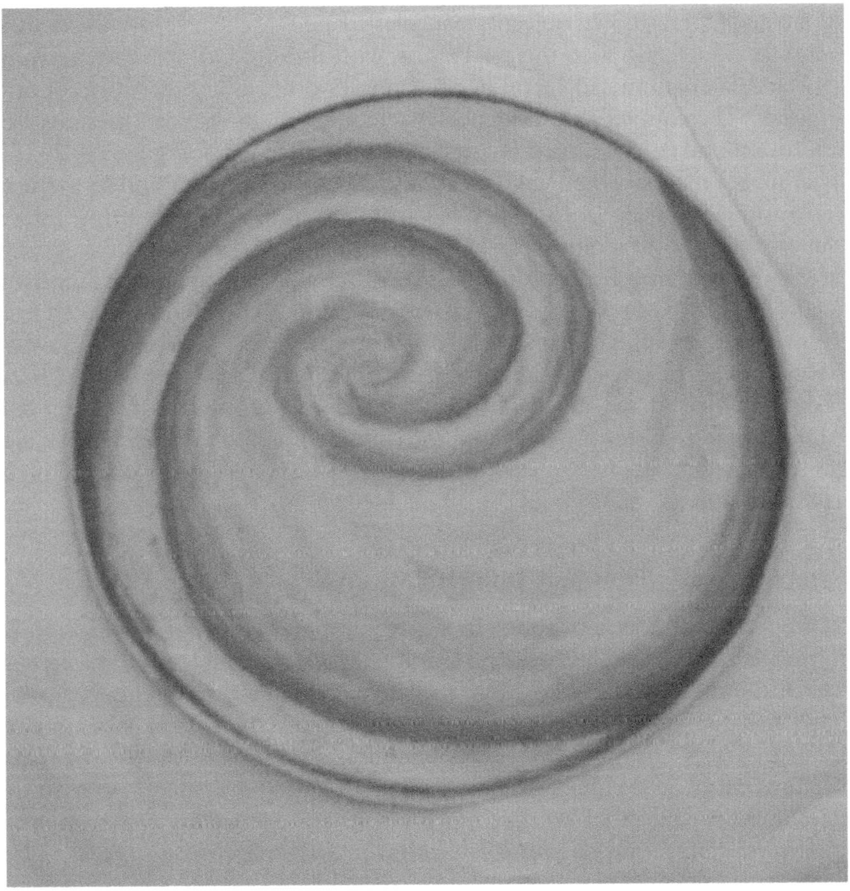

Figure 3.5 Completion art – mandala – 12-year-old male.

In Western psychotherapy, the use of mandalas was first introduced by Carl Jung (1973) who observed that clients became calmer through expressing within a circular frame. Jung regarded mandalas as symbols of wholeness and integration, and also as possible signs from the person's unconscious about a direction for healing in the psyche.

While in traditional cultures, such as Tibetan Buddhism, Navaho Sand Pictures, and Australian aboriginal sand art, mandalas can be complex and highly structured, mandala creation with children in ET is usually not pre-meditated; there is no requirement for them to be planned. Instead, they are "allowed". Usually, such creations flow out spontaneously. Often, however, the emerging image contains a sense of order or balance that can reflect the new internal state of the client. A mandala created by the client can be used at home as a focal point to "hold" connection with themselves between sessions. As a type of "transitional object", mandalas created by clients can support their ongoing connection with their strengths, with therapy and with the therapist.

Mandala creation can be offered as "homework", as another form of self-support. There is reliable evidence that colouring in mandala designs can improve mood (e.g., Curry & Kasser, 2005; Van der Vennet & Serice, 2012). Thai makes mandala "drawing" a useful self-care strategy. Mandala patterns can easily and freely be downloaded from the internet, e.g.: http://www.supercoloring.com/coloring-pages/arts-culture/mandala

Clients suffering from traumatic distress could gain significant improvements in PTSD symptom severity by working through the trauma-related feelings with the creation of mandalas (Henderson at al., 2007). Mandala drawing has been used to support cognitive, socio-emotional and spiritual integration (Young, 2001). Used as an activity for children diagnosed with ADD and ADHD, mandala drawing increased the children's ability to pay attention and resulted in decreased impulsive behaviours (Smitheman-Brown & Church, 1996).

Symbol Work – Show and Tell with Miniatures

"Using symbols is one of the defining characteristics of what it means to be human" (Uttal & Yuan, 2014, p. 295). Children are expected to master the use of numerals, letters and more recently, computer icons. These symbols have culturally attached meanings. Within therapy, metaphor – combining individual symbolic mental imagery communicated through words – has been used to engage and enhance reflection and articulation for decades. With the development of Symbol Work, a more concrete and engaging way to identify internal meanings and communicate about these has arrived.

What Is Symbol Work?

Symbol Work is a way of using miniature figurines for expressing "non-verbal thinking" (Lowenfeld, 2004), for communicating ideas and expressing feelings. It offers a therapeutic modality that generates visual, verbal and spatial exploration through client-generated metaphors. Metaphors expressed through selecting and arranging miniatures can represent both explicit and implicit concerns. When a client has difficulty expressing their dilemmas in words, communicating through images and symbols can provide an alternative language that supports awareness and expression of emotion-laden material about which a client may have limited understanding (Morena, 2008).

Through Symbol Work, clients create visual representations of their world and the nature of relationships they encounter. In addition, Symbol Work provides an avenue for self-expression that is not restricted by language or verbal processing abilities. Symbol Work can help a client understand themselves and their situation, providing markers for a conversation. Symbols can become "magnets for meaning", enhance self-trust and foster the emergence of beneficial self-understanding. At the same time, SW can extend a counsellor's insights about the client and about their experiences, thoughts and feelings (see Figure 3.6).

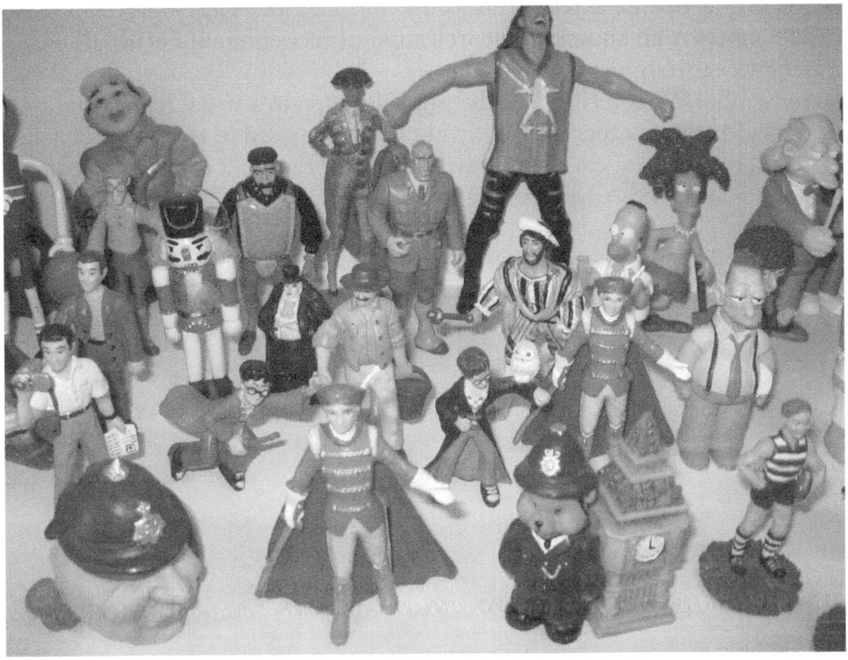

Figure 3.6 Symbol shelf – male figurines.

As you may know, Sandplay Therapy also uses miniatures arranged in sand trays. What distinguishes Symbol Work from Sandplay Therapy is the direction offered by the counsellor. The process evokes a focused, guided, interactive, collaborative communication and understanding. The topic and format are therapist-directed and will usually focus on a specific issue that encourages sharing of internal and external information. Symbol work can also provide an opportunity to three-dimensionally solve a problem.

In ET the projective process of using miniatures to support young clients to reflect, communicate and review their experiences has been highly successful.

The therapist offers suggestions or directs clients to review a shelf of miniatures (most commonly used in non-directive Sandplay Therapy) to create a picture of their concerns. The miniatures become symbols when clients are attracted to them, connect with them and project meaning onto them.

For over 30 years, we have been developing a range of Symbol Work activities. The activities offer a guided way of using miniatures to think, reflect, remember, communicate ideas and, of course, safely express feelings. It offers a therapeutic modality that uses visual and spatial reflection, followed by verbal communication, about client-generated metaphors inspired by the miniatures. These metaphors can represent both explicit and implicit experiences. Symbol Work uses a natural internal projective mechanism. This simply means the psyche makes itself known by identification or recognition of internal states or experiences through external objects.

In Symbol Work a client can be guided to create a visual representation of their world as they experience it. Symbols are also used to represent the nature of relationships they encounter. Symbol Work can be a catalyst for communication and provide markers for a therapeutic conversation (see Figure 3.7).

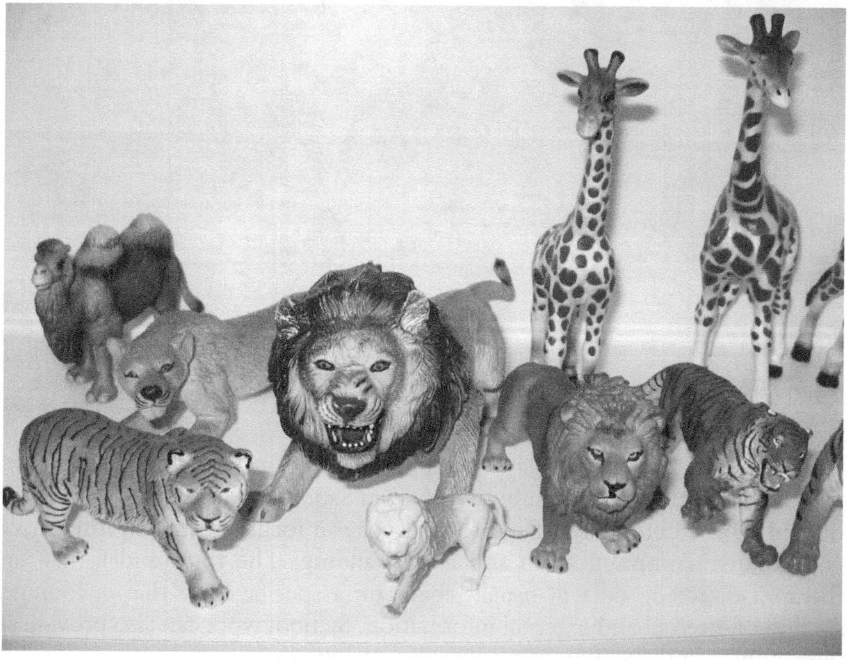

Figure 3.7 Symbol shelf – wild animal figurines.

Guidelines for Symbol Work

- Sit to the side of the client, where you can observe their creation from their viewpoint
- Avoid touching or moving a client's symbols
- Avoid giving a name to the symbols – use only the client's words
- Find out the client's interests or meanings – resist giving your interpretation
- Find what is most interesting to the client and help them trust their own perceptions
- Use your guess about possible meanings to frame open questions
- Resist any temptation to make comments about their choice
- Offer reflection-generating questions that engage the client in exploring their own thoughts, feelings, associations, or meanings
- Remind them they are the expert in themselves, and remember they cannot be wrong
- Invite, rather than instruct
- Listen more than you speak
- Allow silence
- Counsellor returns symbols to shelves after client leaves.

Playful Interactions through Symbol Work

As the world becomes more complicated, so too the lives of children and young clients become more complex and complicated. This means we need many windows through which we can attempt to understand a client – we need to avail ourselves of many views, and support them as they begin to see themselves in different, fresh ways.

Through learning to play and create with the miniatures – that can quickly become symbolic, and hence referred to as "symbols" – the client may come into connection with forgotten or implicit levels of the psyche, including experiences from a pre-verbal time. When distressing or traumatic experiences disrupt a child's development, they may demonstrate heightened stress responses, immobilisation and developmental delays (Badenoch, 2008). Play is considered important in the development of personality and the ability to relate to the world. It contributes to cognitive and social development. Play can reduce stress and activate spontaneity. Spontaneity creates a state where implicit experience can emerge naturally, given the client is equipped with suitable media.

Symbol Work helps overcome conscious and unconscious defences through the fact that it closely resembles play and is non-threatening. By beginning with play and allowing explicit and implicit contents to be projected onto the symbols, the focus is removed from immediate behaviour problems, emotional dysfunction and physical symptoms.

Play that includes projection, metaphor, visual art, symbols and imagination allows vulnerable clients to process difficult issues safely, at their own pace – keeping some issues at a cognitive distance if need be. The use of face-to-face interactions with play-focused methods in counselling makes it possible to navigate high and low-arousal positive states in the nervous system. This happens because the play system is activated in the absence of danger (Kestly, 2016). Active play positively builds resilience through broadening possible behaviours and by providing a context in which the client can learn to manage high-arousal states (Kestly, 2016).

Enhancing Symbol Work Facilitation

In order to provide conditions highly conducive for playful or serious symbol work engagement, a counsellor's participation in transformational learning, having extensive personal experience, professional competence and enjoyment with Symbol Work is a professional requirement. A capacity to create a sense of safety, physically, neurobiologically, emotionally, provides a context that meets the clients' need to feel safe to explore and engage in the process.

As a process, Symbol Work helps gain trust in the client's internal psychological healing mechanisms, the logic of their readiness to determine issues, and timing for therapeutic focus. Our self-awareness and ability to be attentive and empathically attuned help clients feel less isolated as well as support a "corrective experience" in relation to early attachment.

Being comfortable with silence can support clients to relax and take the time they need to feel, reflect and grow in self-awareness. Our capacity for patience and acceptance of the client is crucial, as is our readiness to seek regular practical supervision. In working with miniatures we develop many abilities, such as comfort with "creative doubt", being in an alert and curious state of not knowing. With this, our ability to withhold interpretation of clients' creations, while remaining focused and curious, is central.

Reflective, Self-Discovery and Invitational Questioning

Sensitive facilitation with miniatures and client artwork requires alertness to avoid offering leading questions or making suppositions that incline a client towards an answer they think the counsellor wants to hear. ET activities offer reflective, self-discovery questioning, designed to foster client empowerment;

create more psychological space for implicit material to emerge; empower clients through encouragement of reflection and awareness; and allow the client's own insights to emerge.

Table 3.1 Directive vs Reflective Questioning

Directive leading questions	*Reflective, self-discovery questions*
These questions bring pressure, close down reflection, restrict and limit client responses	These questions bring a sense of freedom, openness, choice and convey interest
Is that wicked witch anything like your mother?	*Would you like to say anything about that symbol?*
Is that lonely elephant very sad?	*Can you say anything more about the elephant? How might it be feeling right now?*
Is that yucky spider making the little rabbit frightened?	*How do you feel about the spider? How do you think the other figures feel about the spider?*
This puppy over here, all alone outside the circle, must feel just like you.	*What do you think that puppy might be thinking and feeling?*

"Why" and "How" Questions

ET uses "how" questions rather than "why" questions. "Why" questions imply that the client should already have a clear reason for what they are doing, and incline the client to stay in a more conscious cognitive mode. "Why" questions can also incline the client to feel confused or inadequate. "How" or more invitational questions generate reflection and self-awareness, and evoke sharing about their experiences.

Table 3.2 Changing why questions to how questions

Why	*How*
Why is it like that?	*How does this feel to you?*
Why is this figure bigger than the others?	*When you look at all the figures you have used, can you say anything about what you notice, or how they feel to you?*
Why did you use so much red in your picture?	*When you look at the colours you have chosen, what stands out? Can you say how you feel when you look at the image?*

Guidelines for Using Art and Symbol in ET

Responding to Clients' Art Creations

Expressive Therapies offers clients a safe way of expressing a wide range of experiences, from heights of positive wellbeing, to inexpressible depths of suffering. ET respects the role of the client and privileges them as the "star of the therapeutic drama" (Duncan et al., 2011), and the interpreter of their experience and creations.

While a therapist may learn much from observing client creations, a non-interpretive approach is used in discussing all art. A client may be invited to interpret or place their own meaning onto the colours, shapes and images they have used. The counsellor, however, always holds back their own emerging ideas. No interpretation of artwork is given by the counsellor. Child and adolescent clients in particular are vulnerable to being affected by inappropriate interpretations, and even with the best intentions, it can be disempowering to provide what to the client seems like an expert opinion. We learn more and have better outcomes from encouraging their reflection on their creation.

While there are several systems that claim to interpret the symbolism of colours, interpretation is avoided and regarded as unhelpful to the process. Although there may be some anecdotal evidence about universal use of colours for say, anger or love, there appears to be no reliable use by children of precise colours for specific feelings. Invite the client to share if they have any comments about colour choices; however, avoid suggesting they should have reasons for their choices. Prize spontaneity.

Confidentiality with drawn (and written) material is paramount. Be aware of any need for safety or privacy for client's artwork. Where would be the safest place for storage of artefacts produced in session? Do you keep a file for your clients containing material produced? Consider who might access the file. Keeping a confidential file within your practice can enable review sessions to guide a client in an overview of their therapeutic journey.

The Physical Environment

Create an area in the consulting room that is uplifting, inspiring, and suggests freedom of expression where being expressive or messy with art materials can happen without constraint. The area ideally inspires with an enticing choice of media. The environment of the counselling room is very important in allowing trust and freedom of expression. For those clients dealing with emotional chaos, a sense of external order is ideal. This would include arrangement of furniture and a general sense of tidiness. In the sensitive state that clients enter a counselling room, beautiful impressions convey a sense of respect and safety. It might be helpful to spend time arranging a special place of beautiful and natural objects (Kamitsis & Simmonds, 2017), perhaps with a candle. It does not take much effort to convey the message that the counselling room is a caring, safe and special place. At the same time, we do not want to create a static, perfect setting that would disincline clients to feel free to express and create.

Client Emotional Safety

Aim to develop rapport as a first step. A sense of calm in the counsellor – and within the room – is important. Ideally, all material and equipment should be ready and accessible prior to the client's arrival. Be aware of any need for safety or privacy for client's artwork. The usual rules about client confidentiality apply equally to their art work. Kalff (2003) in describing the environment best suited for young clients, urged therapists to create a "free and protected space".

Use self-discovery questions when exploring a client's art. Questions ideally support deeper reflection on their creations. Coleman and Farris-Dufrene (1996) emphasise that while a client's art can be interpreted from a variety of theoretical orientations, it is important to understand and privilege the client's interpretation. Similarly, Wadeson (1995, p. 99) says "Interpretation that is not centred in the art-maker's experience may actually interfere with one's more accurate understanding of the art". And we can benefit by reminding ourselves that it is the creative and expressive process that brings change, not the analysis.

Your Empathic Listening

Some clients will be inspired and able to communicate about their experiences through art creation. Some will prefer to remain silent. Accommodate both the extravert and the introvert. Verbal processing of creations is not essential for the art process to be effective. If the client perceives that the counsellor is attentive, present, without judgement, they may be more inclined to just open up and explore previously untried experimentation. Invitational relating demonstrates a respectful attitude towards the client's creations. Invitations encourage reflection, choice and empowerment for clients. Invite them to share their work, never pressure or instruct them to reveal.

Overcoming Client Reticence

As a support to working with clients' negative beliefs about their drawing ability, and to stimulate interest and a flow in expression, it can be useful at times to invite the client to try drawing with their non-dominant hand. Responding to music with drawing may also help generate the creative flow (see page 126). Sometimes sharing your own initial hesitation or even embarrassment about your limited artistic skills will convey empathy and acceptance. For a client, this creates a climate of willingness to experiment and focus on the process, not the product.

PRACTICAL ART & SYMBOL WORK ACTIVITIES

Activity 3.1 Opening Conversation with a New Client: *Supporting Reflection with a Symbol*

The client is invited to browse the shelf of miniatures, then choose the most interesting symbol.

Questions that can guide initial conversations in relation to chosen miniatures:

1. *Would you be able to tell me anything about what you have chosen?*
2. *When you look at it, is there anything that stands out to you?*
3. *Is there a feeling or mood that might go with this symbol?*
4. *Is there anything about it that surprises you?*
5. *Is there anything it reminds you of?*
6. *Are there other ideas that come into your mind when you look at it?*
7. *What might be its main strengths or weaknesses?*
8. *If it could talk, what do you think it would say?*
9. *Are there any others you were attracted to?*

Activity 3.2 Symbol Work Role-Play: *The Most Beautiful Symbol*

This activity helps introduce the symbol collection, supports communicating about self, has an experience of the power of symbol work, builds a positive connection to counselling, and enhances the self-relationship.

- Client selects what to them is the most beautiful or empowering symbol.
- Invite the client to talk about the symbol they selected – what attracted them to it?
- The counsellor will invite the client to hold the symbol and to role-play it. (Briefly explain role-play).
- Ask the following questions slowly, giving the client time to reflect and feel the answer, and then respond.

- Say to the client:
- *Relax as much as you can and take a few steady deep breaths.*
- *For this activity can you pretend you are this beautiful object in your hands?*
- *And I would like to ask the symbol some questions.*
- *If you are comfortable, close your eyes for a moment, let a picture of the symbol come into your mind.* (If the client is not comfortable closing their eyes, eliminate this step).
- *Be interested in how the symbol looks, feels ... what its energy might be like.*
- *Now see if you can imagine yourself becoming this symbol.*

- *Imagine your body changing. You can change your posture if that helps.*
- *Take a moment to imagine the mood, the feelings of this symbol.*
- *Take another full slow breath and feel how it is to be this beautiful thing.*

- The client first imagines self as the symbol then answers these questions, responding with "I" rather than "It".
  1. *Could you tell me what you are?*
  2. *Would you be able to describe what you look like?*
  3. *Could you tell me what is on the inside of you? What you are made of?*
  4. *Do you know where you came from?*
  5. *Do you have a sound or movement? Could you show that?*
  6. *What are your special qualities and strengths?*
  7. *Do you have a special purpose? What are you for?*
  8. *Is there anything you want?*
  9. *Do you have a message for* ....(client's name), *or anything you would like to say to him/her/them?*

After a pause say:

- *When you are ready, take a couple of slow breaths, come back to being yourself, and bring your attention back to this room.*
- *Did you hear that message? Could you say the message?*
- *How does hearing the message feel?*

- After they have had time to discuss their experience, encourage them to:
  - draw something to remind them of the symbol or its feeling or energy
  - write down the message from the symbol, beside the drawing
- Invite them to share how they feel after the activity and to share any insights about how the symbol's message might relate to their life.

Activity 3.3 Symbol Work and Drawing: *Problem-Solving Adventure*

Materials: symbol collection, A3 size paper, crayons, pen, camera.

This activity uses the creation of a story with symbols and drawing, and story-telling, to encourage clients to talk about self and to explore some problem-solving.

1. The Setting

The client is invited to close their eyes, take a few deep breaths, and watch in their imagination:

- *In this activity, I am going to invite you to create a story – an adventure with the symbols and with drawing.*

- *Every story has a starting place.*
- *Where will your story begin? When you say "Once upon a time ..." where will that be?*
- *Will it be on a mountain? In the jungle? Under the ocean? In outer space?*
- *Can you picture this starting place in your mind?*
- *Could you sketch it now? Or could you describe it to me?*

2. Characters in the Story

The client selects five symbols to use in creating the story. Categories:

- most beautiful symbol
- ugliest
- strongest
- weakest
- hero or heroine

They are invited to discuss what they can about each character (symbol), and how each might be feeling at the beginning of the story.

3. Creation and Reflection on the Story

- *This story is an adventure, a quest.*
- *All the characters have to travel together. How will that happen?*
- *Where will it be? Where are they going?*
- *Do they know why they are going? Is there something they are all seeking?*
- *What do you know about each one? What has happened to them just before this story?*
- *How do they relate with each other?*
- *Since they have to stay together, what helps them help each other?*
- *What is the main challenge or difficulty in this adventure?*
- *What are the obstacles?*
- *Are there any helpers?*
- *What will happen at the end?*

4. Story Telling

Client is invited to tell the whole story

5. Integration

Any links between the adventure and the client's life can be discussed.
A photographic record is taken.
The symbols may be drawn onto the page.
The client is invited to record the adventure – as "homework" (where safe to do so).

Activity 3.4 Symbol Work: *My Family, My Life*

Suggested Age Range: from nine years

Materials: Symbol collection available. Drawing paper – A3 size at least – and crayons and pen.

Preparation

1. *Choose your favourite coloured crayon.*
    - *Draw huge imaginary circles in the air, then:*
2. *Draw a large quick circle or oval shape on the paper.*
    - *Call it "My Family/My Life".*
    - *Place a dot at the centre. Write the word "me" next to that dot.*
3. *Take a moment to tune in and feel yourself coming home inside your body.*
    - *Relax as much as you can.*
    - *You could even close your eyes for a moment.*
    - *Take a slow full breath and relax it out.*
4. *Open your mind to a picture of "your family".*
    - *See what comes into your mind. Who or what is "family" for you?*
    - *Can you see them clearly?*
5. *Select from the symbol collection:*
    - *An object that reminds you of you. See if you can let it choose you.*
    - *Don't think too much about it.*
    - *Then can you find something that reminds you of everyone in your image of your family?*
    - *And bring the objects back to the circle you have drawn.*
6. *Place the object for you on the dot at the centre of the circle.*
    - *Do you want to say anything about that?*
7. *See how you feel about these questions as you arrange the other objects on the page:*
    - *How close or distant from you will they be?*
    - *How close or distant from each other will they be?*
    - *How do they connect with each other?*
    - *Are they facing, or turned away from you? from each other?*
    - *Are they inside or outside the circle? Near the circle? Or near the centre?*

8. Discussion questions:

Could you talk about:

- *What you notice when you look at the picture?*
- *How did you arrange the objects?*
- *Each family member and the objects you chose for them?*
- *How does your family connect to each other?*
- *Anyone who is not there on your page?*

9. Client is invited to add some lines that show the connections between the people:

- *strong lines? light lines?*
- *straight lines? curvy lines?*
- *happy lines? unhappy lines?*
- *What colours would the lines be?*

10. Invite the client to reflect on:

- *Is there any way you would like it to be?*
- *Are there any changes you would make?*

As they discuss this, be aware of supporting and encouraging any emotions evoked.

Integration

11. The client can draw the figures onto the page,

- or write the names of the symbols onto the page,
- or take a photo.

12. Allow time for the client to write a few lines about what stands out for them, and their most important feelings or insights from this exercise.

Note:

For adolescent clients it may be more appropriate for them to discern where the dot (in Step 2) should go, to reflect how they feel within the family.

Activity 3.5 Symbol Work, Creativity and Future Focus: *What Would I Like to Do?*

Suggested Age Range: Nine years to adult.

For use with a client towards the end of a series of sessions. This is a resource-building activity, designed to support both intrapersonal reflection and developing goals, directions, inspiration for a future focus.

- Client draws a large circle on a large sheet of paper.
- Invite a preliminary discussion on hobbies, creativity, creative activities the client would like to do or make now and in the future. Encourage them to share any enthusiasms, longings, plans, hopes and dreams.

Expression: The client is asked to select symbols in the following four areas. Invite discussion about the symbol and then invite the client to arrange them in the circle:

1. You Now

- *Could you choose something that goes with you in your life now?* (pause)
- *It would be a symbol that reminds you of yourself or your life now?*
- *Can you tell me anything that attracted you to this figure?*
- *Are there any ways this figure is like you? Or different to you?*

2. A Creative Activity You Like

- *Reflect on a creative activity you would most like to do. This could be something you have not done yet, but would really like to try. Maybe it is something you would like to make?*
- *Could you find a figure or two that goes with this creative activity?*

The client is invited to arrange the symbols in the circle. They are arranged in any way the client feels they relate with each other.

Invite discussion on these symbols. Next, invite the client to add symbols for:

3. What Stops You

- *Is there something stopping you? Is there someone or something that seems to hold you back from doing this activity you want to do?*
- *Is there more of a "No" in you towards this activity, or more of a "Yes"?*

4. Support – What Could Help

- *What – or who – could help you with this creative activity?*
- *Is there anyone who could help you in the future?*

- The client is invited to arrange these additional symbols on the page. Invite the client to arrange them in any way that shows how they relate with each other.
- When the client is satisfied with the arrangement, the counsellor could gently ask questions to help them reflect, such as:
  - *Is there anything you would like to say about this?*
  - *Would you be able to tell me any way this first figure is similar to, or different from you?* (Referring to the first symbol chosen)

    - *How long have you wanted to do this activity?*
    - *How do you feel when you think about this activity?*
    - *Have you ever actually done it?*
    - *Is there any help?*
    - *Are you aware of anything in you that might hold you back from doing it?*
    - *What might the next step be? Would you like to find a symbol for that?*
- They are invited to discuss how they have arranged the symbols.
- The client is encouraged to add colours, lines or words that:
    - add meaning
    - may show connections
    - may show the energies or feelings of the symbols.

Reflection on the Process

The counsellor can offer questions to encourage reflection and self-discovery. Such as:

- *Is there anything that stands out to you when you look at what you have created?*
- *How long have you wanted to do this activity?*
- *Can you imagine how you might feel when you have done it?*

Integration and Strategies

- The client is asked to reflect on and suggest:
    - Any new ideas they have for expressing their creativity.
    - Strategies for working through what gets in the way of doing it.
    - Ideas about finding help or support for this activity – (both client first, then counsellor can make suggestions)
    - One practical step – a starting point – that they could actually take to move towards this creative activity.
- A photographic record may be helpful for the client as reinforcement or motivation for engaging in creative pursuits.

Activity 3.6 Expression Activity: *Emotional Reflection with Drawing and Music*

Materials: Drawing paper and crayons. Divide a large page into four, or use four pages.

Aim: To encourage freedom in the client's drawing expression, and overcoming negative beliefs about drawing (if these exist); to provide opportunities to talk about self and life experiences. This activity works best when the counsellor has first tried the activity for themselves.

Select four tracks of music that express different energies, moods, or emotions.

E.g., strong drumming, gentle flute, militaristic, flowing orchestral, hot rock music, techno, hip-hop, relaxation music (not music with words).

Review clients' attitudes towards drawing.

Part 1: Drawing Music

- Client stands, takes a few deep breaths, closes eyes and opens ears. Counsellor can participate in Part I, along with the client.
- Say: *Listen to the music:*
    - *Can you feel its effect in your body?*
    - *Does your body seem to say YES or NO to the music?*
    - *Does the music make you want to move? Feel free to move if you wish.*
    - *Are there any colours that go with the music?*
    - *How does it make you feel? Does it affect your mood?*
    - *Is there anywhere the music moves inside you?*
    - *Are there any pictures that the music brings to your mind?*
- Play the track of music for about two minutes, no more than 3 minutes.
- *Draw quickly now – use whatever lines, colours, shapes, images you feel go with the music. Don't think much about it, let it happen.*
- *Add a word or two that goes with the colours and mood.*
- Repeat with each music track.
- Discuss: *Would you be willing to share what you have created?*
    - *Was it easy or hard to do?*
    - *Have you ever felt like any of the music we played?*
    - *Did any of the music remind you of anything in your life?*

Part 2: Drawing Feelings

Do not use music for this part of the activity, and do not participate.

- *Relax, lean back or lie down. Take some deep breaths.*

A. *See if you can remember a recent time of fear, or sadness, or hopelessness, or something similar.*

- *Is there any of that feeling in you now? Where would it be in you?*
- *Can you find the colour of that feeling? Let it come into your mind's eye. Is it a pure colour, or mixed? Are there several colours?*
- *Imagine the lines or shapes or pictures that go with that feeling.*

- *Let yourself express again, let it flow out rather than plan it. Let your hand and the crayons do it.* (Pause while they draw.)
- *To the side of your creation, could you write down any thoughts you remember having at that time? Or any words that go with that time?*

B. *Remember a recent time of courage or strength or confidence or hope, or something similar.*

- *Is there any of that feeling in you now? Where would it be in you?*
- *Can you find the colour of that feeling? Let it come into your mind's eye.*
- *Is it a pure colour, or mixed? Are there several colours?*
- *Imagine the lines or shapes or pictures that go with that feeling.*
- *Let yourself express again, whatever you pictured, let it flow, let your hand and the crayons play and express.* (Pause while they draw.)
- *Beside the drawing, could you write down any thoughts you remember having at that time? Or any words that go with that time?*

- Discuss these two drawings now. E.g.:
    - *Would you like to talk about what you have drawn?*
    - *Is one drawing more interesting?*
    - *Would you like to say more about the colours and lines you have used?*
    - *Did you find the feelings inside you? Or could you remember where they were?*
    - Discuss ways to use drawing as an emotional stress reduction strategy, and any times or circumstances when this might be beneficial.
- Discuss how they feel about art and drawing now.

Follow-Up Option

If there is a need to process emerging feelings further:

- Invite the client to choose emotionally specific music to go with the feelings identified
- briefly listen to the music together to assess its suitability
- invite them to stand and:
    - listen to the music
    - move with it – or imagine moving to the music
    - draw several quick drawings in response
- Sit: How do you feel now? Remember any times when you may have felt a bit like this, and discuss.

Other Reflection Options

A: A recent time of frustration, annoyance or anger
   A recent time of peace, calmness, relaxation or stillness.
B: A recent time when things felt boring, dull or useless
   A recent time of excitement, aliveness, energy or happiness.

Activity 3.7 Process Art – 1: *Drawing Out Troubles*

Materials: Large selection of coloured crayons available, large art pad or long roll of drawing paper. Availability of a range of coloured papers may also be useful.

Aim: An emotional release activity using continuous drawing of reactions to help reduce emotional stress.

1. The client is invited to focus on a reaction to a troubling issue they have identified.

The client is guided to tune in to self, to connect as fully as possible with the reaction

- imagining what colour, or colours, go with their feelings
- imagining what lines feel right to show their feelings
- and to begin using colours, lines, shapes to depict the feelings.

As they progress with the process art, keep inviting them to:

- tune in to self, to the current feelings,
- look over the range of crayons to see what colour or colours feel right to represent the internal experience at the moment.

2. They are encouraged to start drawing across the page and then down the page, in rows, columns or free-style. Offer options. Encourage the expression to be spontaneous and continuous. The client is encouraged to keep drawing, without thinking too much about the result, using as many pages – or as much paper – as they wish.

- They are invited to reflect on what sorts of lines would best show their feelings, and to:
  - keep producing these lines
  - at the same time observing if those particular lines still seem to show their feelings.
  - Help the client participate in the activity as an experiment, making it clear there is no "correct" way to do it.

3. The counsellor may offer supportive suggestions and questions, such as:

- *Notice if you want to draw faster or slower.*
- *Check inside, how does it feel to do this?*
- *Is there more of that? It's your experiment! You can try out all sorts of different colours, lines and shapes!*

- *Has the feeling inside you changed? How could you show that?*
- *What colours and lines feel right just now?*
- *Are there any words you would like to add that go with that?*
- *Are there any words that want to jump out onto the page?*
- *Do you want to continue? You can stop at any time whenever it feels finished.*

If the client seems "stuck", you could say: *Maybe tune in to yourself again for a moment and then start again – with fresh lines and shapes.*

 - *What colours and lines would go next?*
 - *What colours and lines would you like to end with?*

4. When the client feels finished with the action of drawing, invite them to stand up, stretch, shake, take a few deep breaths, then ask:

- *Are there any pages or areas of the drawing that show how your body would like to move? Could you try that out now?*

5. *Review what you have done:*

- *Is it how you would like to leave it?*
- *Does it feel finished?*
- *Is there anything more you would like to add?*

6. Questions to support the review of the process could be offered when the client is ready, e.g.:

- *Is there anything you could tell me about the feeling inside you now?*
- *Looking back over what you have created – what do you notice? Is there anything that stands out?*
- *Is there a colour, shape, word or picture that you would like to end with now?*

7. Integration

- *Could you find some words that go with: How the activity felt? And how you feel now?*
- *How do you want to finish with the drawing(s)?*
- *Does anything need to happen now? Are there any action steps that would help with the problem?*
- *Walk around the room for a moment, let your arms swing free, let your body relax as you walk.*

Activity 3.8 Process Art – 2: *Exploring Feelings with Drawing, Images and Words*

Materials: large drawing paper (A3 size), crayons, pen, journal, miniatures, Feeling Words Lists

Preparation: Divide a large page into four segments – with lines through the middle vertically and horizontally. Prepare another page with a mandala circle.

Aim: To develop emotional literacy, to build the ability to identify, express and process emotion.

Provide a brief overview of the activity. Confirm that the client has the option to keep their creation private.

Process: Client is guided to find a comfortable way to sit and relax as much as possible, then tune into their body.

- They are asked to scan through the body and identify any areas where they find feelings, even something that doesn't seem to have a name.
- After a minute or two with internal focus, the client indicates which feeling is clearest or strongest, one that stands out from the others, or may be troublesome.
- Invite the client to identify where it is, and if possible, what the feeling is, but it is OK if they cannot name it. Then they relax and refocus on the feeling again.

1. Colours

- While focusing on the feeling, the client is invited to "ask the feeling" what colours it would use to express itself. How would it show itself with colours? It could be one colour, several colours, light or dark colours.
- These colours are then shaded into the first segment of the page.

2. Lines

Client relaxes again, takes a deep breath and tunes in to the feeling again.

The client asks the feeling what type of lines would best show how it feels: E.g., straight lines, sharp jagged lines, smooth curving lines, fat lines, thin lines, broken lines, lines with sharp edges or lines with fuzzy edges?

These are drawn into the second segment.

3. Image

The client is invited to relax again and tune into the feeling.

They ask the feeling if there is a picture of something that goes with how it feels, e.g., *Is the feeling like a place? Or a landscape? The weather or a plant? a tree? An animal? a bird? a fish? Or an insect? Is it like something built by people?*

These are quickly sketched into the third segment on the page. Mention that there is no need for drawing skills.

Alternatively, if pictorial representation is troublesome for the client, they can choose miniatures from the symbol collection.

4. Words

The client is invited to relax again and tune into the feeling.

The client is invited to ask the feeling if there are any words, statements or questions it wants to express. If it could speak or write, what would it say?

Suggest: *There might be just a few words, or lots of them! You can write them big or small. More words might come into your mind once you begin. Sometimes words may come quickly, sometimes they may take a while, sometimes there may not be any. See what you find, and you can use the Feeling Words Lists to help.*

Responses are written on the fourth segment.

Integration: Stand, stretch, take a deep breath, then sit again.

The client is invited to take some time to tune into the feeling again and examine:

- if it feels the same, or
- if there has been any change:

~ *It could be a small change or it could be a big change. See what you notice.*

Discussion is invited on:

- How they feel now?
- Any changes they noticed during the activity?
- Is there any movement they would like to make that goes with the feeling?
- Any possible causes of the feeling?
- How the feeling relates to their life; e.g., is it a frequent feeling? Or unusual?
- Is there anything external that needs to change? Any steps to take?

Completion Mandala

- Client is guided to tune in again, to scan their whole body, then focus on the area of the feeling(s).
- *Let the feeling now use your hand, these crayons, and draw whatever it wants in the mandala circle.*
- Does the client wish to say anything about the final creation?

References

Badenoch, B. (2008). *Being a brain-wise therapist: A practical guide to interpersonal neurobiology*. W. W. Norton & Company.

Berman, H. (2001). Children and war: Current understandings and future directions. *Public Health Nursing, 18*(4), 243–252.

Boehm, K., Cramer, H., Staroszynski, T., & Ostermann, T. (2014). Arts therapies for anxiety, depression, and quality of life in breast cancer patients: A systematic review and meta-analysis. *Evidence-Based Complementary and Alternative Medicine, 2014*(1), 103297.

Cavazos, K. R. (2012). *Therapists' perspective on the effectiveness of art therapy*. California State University.

Cohen-Yatziv, L., & Regev, D. (2019). The effectiveness and contribution of art therapy work with children in 2018. What progress has been made so far? A systematic review. *International Journal of Art Therapy, 24*(3), 100–112.

Coleman, V. D., & Farris-Dufrene, P. M. (1996). *Art therapy and psychotherapy - Blending two therapeutic approaches*. Accelerated Development.

Cooper, M., Di Malta, G., Knox, S., Oddli, H. W., & Swift, J. K. (2023). Patient perspectives on working with preferences in psychotherapy: A consensual qualitative research study. *Psychotherapy Research*. Advance online publication.

Cooper, M., & McLeod, J. (2011). Person-centered therapy: A pluralistic perspective. *Person-Centered & Experiential Psychotherapies, 10*(3), 210–223.

Curry, N. A., & Kasser, T. (2005). Can coloring mandalas reduce anxiety? *Art Therapy, 22*(2), 81–85.

Duncan, B. L., Miller, S. D., & Sparks, J. A. (2011). *The heroic client: A revolutionary way to improve effectiveness through client-directed, outcome-informed therapy*. John Wiley & Sons.

Eaton, L. G., Doherty, K. L., & Widrick, R. M. (2007). A review of research and methods used to establish *art* therapy as an effective treatment method for traumatized children. *Arts in Psychotherapy, 34*(3), 256–262.

Fincher, S. (2009). *The mandala workbook. A creative guide for self-exploration, balance, and well-being*. Shambhala Publications.

Gilroy, A. (2006). *Art therapy, research and evidence-based practice*. Sage.

Gladding, S. T. (1998). *Counseling as an art: The creative arts in counseling*. American Counseling Association.

Grant, J., & Crawley, J. (2002). *Transference and projection: Mirrors to the self*. Open University Press.

Henderson, P., Mascaro, N., Rosen, D., & Skillern, T. (2007). Empirical study on the healing nature of mandalas. *Psychology of Aesthetics, Creativity and the Arts, 1*(3), 148–154.

Joschko, R., Klatte, C., Grabowska, W. A., Roll, S., Berghöfer, A., & Willich, S. N. (2024). Active visual art therapy and health outcomes: a systematic review and meta-analysis. *JAMA Network Open, 7*(9), e2428709-e2428709.

Jung, C. G. (1973). *Mandala symbolism*. Bollingen Series.

Kalff, D. M. (2003). *Sandplay. A psychotherapeutic approach to the psyche*. Temenos Press.

Kamitsis, I., & Simmonds, J. G. (2017). Using resources of nature in the counselling room: Qualitative research into ecotherapy practice. *International Journal for the Advancement of Counselling, 39*, 229–248.

Kapitan, L. (2011). *An introduction to art therapy research.* Routledge.
Kestly, T. A. (2016). Presence and play: Why mindfulness matters. *International Journal of Play Therapy, 25*(1), 14–23.
Kramer, E. (1958). *Art therapy in a children's community.* Thomas.
Lazarus, A. A. (1982). *Personal enrichment through imagery* (Audiotape). BMA Audio Cassettes.
Lowenfeld, M. (2004). *Understanding children's sandplay: Lowenfeld's world technique.* Liverpool University Press.
Lusebrink, V. B. (1990). *Imagery and visual expression in therapy.* Plenum Press.
Malchiodi, C. A. (2005). *Expressive therapies.* Guilford Press.
McNiff, S. (1992). *Art as medicine. Creating a therapy of the imagination.* Shambhala.
McNiff, S. (2004). *Art heals: How creativity heals the soul.* Shambhala.
McNiff, S. (2012). Art-based methods for art therapy assessment. In A. Gilroy, R. Tipple, & C. Brown (Eds.), *Assessment in art therapy* (pp. 66–80). Routledge.
Millard, E., Cardona, J., Fernandes, J., Priebe, S., & Carr, C. (2021). I know what I like, and I like what I know: Patient preferences and expectations when choosing an arts therapies group. *The Arts in Psychotherapy, 75*, 101829.
Morena, G. D. (2008). Midwives of consciousness: Supervising sandplay and expressive art therapists. In H. S. Friedman & R. Rogers Mitchell (Eds.), *Supervision of sandplay therapy* (pp. 215–221). Routledge.
Nabarro, M. (2005). Feast of colour. In D. Kalmanowitz & B. Lloyd (Eds.), *Art therapy and political violence with art, without illusion* (pp. 81–82). Routledge.
Oaklander, V. (1988). *Windows to our children - A gestalt therapy approach to children and adolescents.* Real People Press.
Oster, G. D., & Montgomery, S. S. (1996). *Clinical uses of drawings.* Jason Aronson Inc.
Payne, H. L. (1993). *A handbook of inquiry in the arts therapies: One river, many currents.* Jessica Kingsley Publications.
Rothschild, B. (2000) *The body remembers: The psychophysiology of trauma and trauma treatment.* W. W. Norton and Company.
Skovholt, T. M., Morgan, J. I., & Negron-Cunningham, H. (1989). Mental imagery in career counselling and life planning: A review of research and intervention methods. *Journal of Counseling and Development, 67*, 287–292.
Smitheman-Brown, V., & Church, R. P. (1996). Mandala drawing: Facilitating creative growth in children with A.D.D. or A.D.H.D. *Art Therapy: Journal of the American Art Therapy Association, 13*(4), 252–260.
Uttal, D. H., & Yuan, L. (2014). Using symbols: Developmental perspectives. *Wiley Interdisciplinary Reviews: Cognitive Science, 5*(3), 295–304.
Van Der Vennet, R., & Serice, S. (2012). Can coloring mandalas reduce anxiety? A replication study. *Art Therapy, 29*(2), 87–92.
Wadeson, H. (1995). *The dynamics of art therapy.* John Wiley and Sons, Inc.
Wolpe, J. (1958). *Psychotherapy by reciprocal inhibition.* Stanford University Press.
Young, A. J. (2001). Mandalas. Circling the square in education. *Encounter: Education for Meaning and Social Justice, 14*(3), 25–33.

4 Stringing Words Together

Therapeutic Writing

Introduction to Therapeutic Writing

An important part of therapy is helping young people "find" their voice, their sense of authenticity and self-authority. Disclosure in the form of the spoken word has long been considered beneficial and widely used in counselling (Mugerwa & Holden, 2012). Language has generally been afforded the privilege of being the primary healing resource in Western counselling practices. Therapeutic writing has been found to have the potential to heal – psychologically and physiologically (Mugerwa & Holden, 2012).

The ET style of therapeutic writing activities evolved in response to client needs and our personal experiences within the client role. We created formats and adapted from the literature forms of creating an imagined autobiography, writing about a particular life event, reflective writing, using Self-Discovery Worksheets, sentence starters, process writing and completion summaries, exploring client-generated imaginary narratives and writing with guiding questions to enhance and record somatic awareness. Therapeutic writing activities can include story construction, use of diaries, journals, letters, poetry and lyrics. We have found the most popular form of therapeutic writing, and most frequently used, is offering sentence stems or sentence starters. These act as catalysts for self-reflection and in-session communication. Writing about stressful events can be an indirect way of contacting experiences that may underlie a reluctance towards re-experiencing. Therapeutic writing can be a process through which a client can re-contact, reflect, ventilate and integrate experience.

Therapeutic writing is suitable for young people who feel comfortable using this medium or who have some affinity with a verbal/linguistic intelligence. Writing is a resource that can clarify thoughts, beliefs and emotions. It can also elicit a sense of vulnerability and exposure for some young clients. In terms of therapy, this vulnerability is actually a strength. The aim is to allow vulnerability to be an active resource. In a life where free expression may not have a safe space, writing a personal narrative or notes about personal experiences can provide a source of quiet empowerment.

DOI: 10.4324/9781003671879-4

The verbal-linguistic intelligence (Gardner, 1983) has been at the core of western psychotherapy since Freud adopted the term "the talking cure" (Freud, 1920). This intelligence is used extensively in verbal therapy and is ideal for clients who think and learn through spoken and written words, have the ability to memorise facts, fill in workbooks, respond to written tasks and enjoy reading. However, for clients with lesser verbal-linguistic ability, offering other modalities and intelligences may be essential. The verbal/linguistic intelligence clearly underlies traditional verbal exchanges in therapy, in therapeutic writing (Pearson & Wilson, 2009; Wright & Chung, 2001), the use of journals (Progoff, 1992), bibliotherapy (Pardeck & Markward, 1995), and in poetry therapy (Bolton & Ihanus, 2011).

Trusting a client's resources sufficiently to afford them a sense of control in a session supports their ability to more readily let go of defensiveness when they wish. This appears to greatly enhance the therapeutic alliance. However, the use of writing for therapeutic outcome has been linked to a range of aspects of wellbeing. These include enhanced immune functioning, improved liver enzyme function, reducing the frequency of health centre visits, and greater effectiveness in coping with job loss and regaining employment (Kenardy & Piercy, 2006; Pennebaker & Seagal, 1999).

Therapeutic writing assists a client's process of selecting what to focus on in sessions. At the same time, a client experiences the capacity to control the pace of disclosure. Providing writing activities can act as a stimulus for more creative, resourceful problem-solving (Riordan, 1996). One of the fundamental tenets of our approach to ET is that a client presents for therapy with internal resources to deal with their problems, as noted by Bohart and Tallman (1996). Each client has a different story, a different experience and a different way of communicating their narrative. To enhance therapeutic change, the therapist's role is to make sure there are sufficient resources, ideas, scaffolds, experiential techniques, space and time for the client.

In an ET approach, a younger client can benefit greatly from support to engage in a process of recording (Oaklander, 1978). Oaklander described a number of ways to engage young clients in using words and writing to enhance their sense of inner strength. For example, completing sentences, writing about opposites, as well as writing longer essays (when age appropriate) that reflect desires, needs, inclinations and emotions.

Evidence Base for Therapeutic Writing

The successful use of writing as a therapeutic tool has been well documented (e.g., Connolly Baker & Mazza, 2004; Kenardy & Piercy, 2006; Pennebaker & Seagal, 1999; Waters, 2002; Wright & Chung, 2001). Evidence from decades of research shows a positive impact from expressive writing in many domains of physical and psychological health, particularly in the aftermath of trauma (Peterkin & Prettyman, 2009). Client-constructed narratives can be regarded as "causally connected events that provide the context for framing and interpreting experience" (Peterkin & Prettyman, 2009, p. 81). A young client may present confused narratives and have interpreted events in an unproductive way; learning how they made sense of events and helping them evolve more realistic and cohesive self-narratives becomes vital. In trauma recovery, MacCurdy (2000) notes, following stressful experiences, verbalising or re-narrating fragmented traumatic experiences may help reconnect "affect with cognition, image with narrative".

Studies have illuminated multiple benefits of therapeutic writing in relation to a range of medical conditions (Mugerwa & Holden, 2012), including: Reduced anxiety and depressive symptoms among those with maladaptive rumination; reduction in depressive symptoms, trauma-related cognitions and general behavioural problems in children with post-traumatic stress disorder. The value of therapeutic writing in a number of important areas was also demonstrated by Haertl and Ero-Phillips (2019), who found it useful to support perspective taking, to develop enhanced understanding of self and others. Additionally, they found the spiritual nature of writing supported the promotion of health and healing.

Burton and King (2004) found there were health benefits from just 2 minutes of written expression, two days in a row. In essence, this short writing process may have allowed participants with a trauma history to harness the power of "unfinished business" to accelerate closure and resolution. Analyses revealed that in general even just 2 minutes of writing about a trauma or a positive topic were, indeed, experienced as beneficial. Research on therapeutic writing also highlights that clients may initially experience immediate increases in uncomfortable feelings, but gain long-term benefits.

Therapeutic writing, within a CBT programme, with children between 8 and 18 years who experienced a range of single and recurrent traumatic experiences, was effective in reducing post-traumatic stress disorder symptoms, depressive symptoms, trauma-related cognitions and general behavioural problems, with effects still in place at a six month follow up (Van der Oord et al., 2010).

Drawing, writing and mutual story-telling techniques were used as part of a five-day programme with children with high anxiety levels, hospitalised for cancer treatment (Altay et al., 2017). The children were asked to draw a picture of a hospitalised child and write a story about their drawing, with mutual storytelling after drawing and writing. These methods were found to be effective in helping children articulate their views as well as reducing their anxiety.

Therapeutic writing can enable clients to explore narratives from various perspectives, such as reflection on values, feelings and identity; to use metaphors for issues that may be too distressing to articulate directly; and to enable clearer self-observations for description and reflection (Bolton & Ihanus, 2011). More recently, Deveney and Lawson (2022) found that after four weekly writing tasks about a personal difficulty, participants reported significant benefits, such as improvements to their processing of emotional difficulty, and increased positive mood and wellbeing.

Positive Writing

The dawn of an expanded focus, since around the 2000s, on the positive in psychology generally, and in therapeutic writing – i.e., happiness, actualisation, wellbeing – encourages us to turn attention towards deepening experiences of satisfaction, gratitude, awe, wellbeing. Expressive writing – writing about traumatic, stressful or emotional events – often leads to improvements in physical and psychological health in non-clinical and clinical populations (Baikie et al., 2012). The benefits of positive writing have also been verified in more recent studies (e.g., Hoult et al., 2025).

Therapeutic writing may involve short-term focused "positive" writing for mood elevation. Other therapeutic writing approaches aim at longer-term outcomes involving reframing negative thoughts, gaining insight and broadening cognitive focus (Ross, 2017). In another study of positive writing (Round et al., 2022), participants completed either three consecutive days of positive writing or writing about a more neutral topic online, 20 minutes per day. For participants in the positive writing condition, there was significantly less anxiety compared to the neutral writing condition.

Youth who were participants in the child welfare and juvenile justice systems in the USA, exhibited significant gains in resilience compared to a control group, when they took part in the WRITE ON (Writing and Reflecting on Identity to Empower Ourselves as Narrators) program (Greenbaum & Javdani, 2017). All participants in a study by Baikie, Geerligs and Wilhelm (2012) showed significant improvements over time on mental health and some physical health outcomes. When expressive and positive writing groups were combined, the resulting "emotional writing group" showed significantly lower scores on the DASS stress subscale. In another study, 90 undergraduates were randomly assigned to write about either an intensely positive experience or a control topic for 20 minutes each day for three consecutive days (Burton & King, 2004). Mood measures were taken before and after writing. Three months later, measures of health centre visits for illness were obtained. Writing about the intensively positive experiences was associated with enhanced positive mood; and was associated with significantly fewer health centre visits, compared to the control group.

A narrative review (Ruini & Mortara, 2022) searched scientific databases and analysed essential studies, academic books and journal articles where writing therapy was applied. The review aimed to describe and summarise the use of writing therapy across a variety of psychotherapies. The results showed positive therapeutic effects on symptoms and distress, but it also indicated that writing can promote psychological wellbeing. The use of writing can be a standalone treatment, or easily integrated as a supplement in other therapeutic approaches.

Poetry Therapy

Research on poetry therapy reached its highest levels between 1999 and 2010, primarily in the USA (Heimes, 2011). Poetry therapy has been found to aid emotional regulation, alleviate psychological suffering and restore balance (Heimes, 2011), having been applied to support anxiety disorders, depression and schizophrenia. In somatic medicine, poetry therapy has been used to support coping with illness and improvement in quality of life. One aim of using poetry in the psychological healing process is to bring forward a response from the client that will help them become more active in the therapeutic process (Koppman, 2001).

The first empirical studies focused on group therapies and used inpatient and other institutional settings as test sites (McCulliss, 2011). Back in 1979, Edgar compared a poetry therapy group to a conventional therapy group in a hospital for schizophrenic patients. The study showed improvement in attitudes, and more patients were discharged home. Kloser (2013) found poetry therapy had a contributing effect to positive youth development (e.g., promoting self-expression, self-esteem, self-identification, decision-making and team cohesion, motivating for success, and aiding in cognitive processes). From a review of the literature, Diana et al (2024) recommend poetry as a medium of counselling to reduce adolescents' problems, such as lack of confidence, low self-esteem, depression, stress and anxiety.

Not only poetry creation, but also reading of poetry can be helpful. For adolescents, in a school setting, reading poetry was effective for improving self-concept (Shahrabady et al., 2021). Writing and reading poetry helps clinicians, students and clients give voice to situations that are important to them (Raingruber, 2004).

Metaphor in Counselling

Metaphor allows the therapist to bypass client reservations and gently build a foundation for opening communication indirectly, before being more direct about challenging topics. In 1990, Combs and Freedman recommended the use of metaphor in counselling and referred to the smallest units of metaphor as "symbols" – words, objects and mental images dense with meaning. They describe how a symbol can generate powerful associations. In ET it is the multiple associations that internal or external images can carry for a client that heighten the effectiveness of the process and lead to acknowledgement and recognition of important issues and enhanced clarity.

The use of metaphor encourages active mental searching on the part of a client. Mental searching can open access to internal resources, stimulate new associative pathways, elicit client creativity and engagement in therapy. Imagery can enhance a client's motivation for active involvement in the healing process (Lusebrink, 1990). Imagery can strengthen the link between body, mind and emotion. Metaphors can provide distancing and externalisation, which can make issues easier to work with. Freeman (1997) found that young people prefer to communicate about problems obliquely, in metaphor or in play, and that externalising language encourages this.

Metaphors may play a significant role in supporting at least five change processes in counselling (Lyddon et al., 2001). These are: Relationship building, accessing and symbolising client emotions, uncovering and challenging clients' assumptions, working with client resistance and introducing new frames of reference.

Therapeutic Writing Methods

Among therapeutic writing methods, there are primarily open-ended writing tasks, such as expressing reflections in a journal, and programmed or guided tasks. Some research suggests positive outcomes are associated with more structured writing programmes, while others point to benefits from unstructured journaling (Peterkin & Prettyman, 2009).

Therapeutic writing offers a tool for developing self-awareness. The process can include recalling, reviewing, selecting and writing down, and then commenting on thoughts, feelings, attitudes, sensations, behaviours, dreams, hopes and plans. This can be a prelude to more open communication in therapy, as well as a therapeutically valuable process in itself. Regular therapeutic writing or journaling can also be used to enhance and record somatic awareness, which in turn can lead to enhanced emotional awareness. For example, Progoff's (1992) "Dialogue with Body", in which a client writes to and from a body part, or somatic aspect of self. It can support processing of issues about counselling and adjustment to the counsellor and counselling environment. Reflection and writing can help a client gain clarity and access issues needing attention. It is an alive process that, whether structured or unstructured, is most effective if it remains flexible and responsive to moment-to-moment changes.

Writing in therapy can take a variety of formats. A client can use written language in personal letters, diaries, statements of feelings, lists of opposites, poetry, short drama dialogues, or autobiographical or time-line reviews. Media can be combined so that drawing, writing and using miniatures (symbol work) come together in one activity to provide a richly textured representation of problems being discussed, as well as concretising insights and emerging plans. All these formats can be utilised to summarise a client's discoveries and to describe, chronicle and consolidate their progress (Payne, 2006).

In ET, therapeutic writing is offered through three broad approaches:

1. **Process Writing**: Writing continuously and spontaneously to work through reactivity, where the process, not the product, is a central focus. Self-inhibition of negative emotions is thought to lead to continuous autonomic arousal and poorer health (Pennebaker & Beall, 1986).

Process writing offers an antidote. Written work offers a space for safe, open expression of feelings, thoughts and insights. These can change or transform during the writing and become clearer. The uncensored flow of written words means the process can also be used by clients for private emotional regulation. Review of spontaneous written expression can help make sense of emotional pain.

2. **Reflective Writing**: Is used to gather together, review, ponder, reflect and make sense of experience. During reflective writing, the mind is focussed to recollect and connect feelings with attitudes and experiences. These writing tasks can focus on:

   - Clarifying decision making. (For this, divide a page, list the pros and cons, the Yes and No options);
   - Dialoguing with parts of self, especially useful when clients appear confused, and/or may be torn between two apparent opposites. For example:
   - *I want to … I don't want to …*
   - *My optimistic part says … My pessimistic part says …*
   - Recording observations and experiences for later reflection, for example using a thought diary, setting up aims or plans and recording outcomes;
   - Reviewing the past to make sense of the present, to discern if any past experiences strongly influence present behaviours and cognition.

3. **Completion Writing**: is an integrative step, to summarise, to use left hemisphere functions to support closure after significant right hemisphere emotion functioning. The activity of sentence completion aids integration; it brings experiences together and supports meaning-making. Writing tasks can spontaneously or deliberately focus on:

   - A review of experiences (within a counselling session)
   - Clarifying intended action steps and future directions
   - Identifying and reinforcing the availability of support
   - Practising gratitude, savouring and recording what has been welcomed and appreciated.

Nine Therapeutic Writing Methods

The range of structured therapeutic writing methods and scaffolding used in ET includes the use of:

1. Topic headings, e.g.:
   - *Write three words that go with: Being at home; being at school; being with friends; having fun. etc.*
2. Prompts or sentence starters, e.g.:
   - *What I really want is …*
   - *What I don't want is …*

3. Questions as catalysts for reflection and response, e.g.:
   - *If I were a counsellor, I would ask my clients about ...*
   - *If I were a parent, I would never ...*
4. Client's own summary of topics of interest as prompts or categories for reflection, e.g.:
   - *Playing soccer*
   - *Being in class with Mr X*
   - *Avoiding enemies*
5. Creating simple forms of poetry, e.g., haiku.
6. Stream-of-consciousness writing – no structure, no stopping, no reflection. Eliminating the need to carefully consider, shape and edit writing allows a very direct, intimate glimpse into self.
7. Scrapbook work or collage: This can include cutting, arranging and pasting of printed headlines and images. These intuitive and spontaneous creations, which do not need to make sense during the creation phase, allow free association, projection onto the page of internal experiences and support releasing uncomfortable emotions.
8. Writing stimulated by visuals includes a selection of interesting, relevant miniatures or photographs to encourage articulation.
9. Completion of worksheets that invite self-reflection and self-discovery through the invitation to use words for metaphor, with additional use of colour, imagery and symbols.

Have available a range of coloured pencils and pens and coloured papers. Clients make choices about media preferences that represent different feelings, aspects of self, differing or opposite perspectives.

Offering a varied range of activities to stimulate or catalyse reflection and communication is helpful (O'Brien & Burnett, 2000). When a client can articulate thoughts, feelings and conflicts, they feel more emotionally satisfied, gain a clearer sense of identity and more easily identify and accept internal direction (Case & Dalley, 1992; Dalley et al., 1993; Landgarten, 1981; Oster & Gould, 1987; Rubin, 1978).

Journal Writing

Journaling can be a very helpful process to assist in generating and documenting personal growth. The emphasis is on the word "process" This means the writing comes alive and emerges from realisations in the moment. This self-knowledge contributes to the ability to discover more creative choices in life. It also means that, as self-observation is underway, internal changes emerge as writing progresses.

Journals act like an internalised counsellor. In journals, clients can confide, capture self-talk for review, dialogue with and clarify parts of themselves, e.g.: *a resentful part can talk to a pleaser part. A dragon part can talk to a princess.* Private secrets can be confidentially acknowledged. Hopes, dreams and longing can be acknowledged. Journal techniques can mix prose writing, sentences, phrases, words, sketches, mind maps, collage and photographs. Younger children can use drawings, body outlines and photographs of symbol work as visual records in their "special book". Parents must respect the person's privacy.

Journal writing is a way of developing a connection with, and interest in, the internal world. The journal can mark the crossing of a threshold between inner and outer worlds, the private and public selves. The aim is increased self-other communication and self-awareness. Today's technology offers speed and accuracy in writing. However, research has shown that writing by hand has advantages. Handwriting activates a broader network of brain regions, such as regions associated with emotional processing and self-awareness (Marano, et al., 2025). While for some children the comfort of a screen may be attractive, we recommend offering pens, pencils and paper.

Clients need the option to keep journals safe and private, so writing can be honest and uncensored. This is important when young clients live in an environment where it is not acceptable or safe to speak openly about their truth. If the home environment does not provide safety and respect for the privacy of journals, can they be stored with the counsellor and used prior to, during, and immediately after sessions? In responding to a client's sharing of written work, respect is paramount, with no judgement on content, style, spelling, grammar or handwriting.

As a medium for reflection, journal writing provides space to process reactions and can act as preparation for clear communication with others. Journals are private, so expression can be truthful and poetic. Journals allow the profound, sensitive, vulnerable, poetic or spiritual to emerge. Some clients may feel they can use poetic words and phrases to clarify deep feelings but may be sensitive about revealing this part of self. They might avoid or hide this part of themselves; however, in their journal, it can come to life. In abusive, unsafe or non-supportive contexts, it might seem easier to keep hidden these aspects of self. Allowing the emergence of poetic or symbolic language is comforting and assists the client's self-development and sense of worth.

Ideally, the journal itself is attractive and regarded as special. It calls for careful attention to the task at hand. The journal itself can be a device, a metaphor for the inner world and the therapeutic journey. A journal can be used:

- as a dynamic process, not merely as a way of making a static record
- at the conclusion of sessions to support integrative focus on what has happened
- as a support for understanding and reflection
- to record dreams, in preparation for future exploration in sessions.

Get the Most from Using a Journal

- Whatever you write is right! You can't do it wrong.
- Try to write for a few minutes every day or every week.
- Write by hand.
- Set a regular reflection and writing time each day or each week.
- Find a special, private, space that could encourage writing.
- Keep writing materials easily accessible.
- Experiment: Does structure or free form work best?
- Don't worry about spelling, or what others might think about what is written.
- Find a safe and private place to keep the journal.
- Decide if you plan to keep your work private or consider who you might like to share it with.

THERAPEUTIC WRITING ACTIVITIES

Activity 4.1 Introduction to Using Sentence Starter Worksheet Activities

Age Range: From 10 years.

Materials: Pen, *Expressive Writing Sentence Starter Worksheet*

Aim: Writing prompts (sentence starters) are designed to generate reflection and flow in expression and support clients in recognising their boundaries and preferred topics. The technique gives permission for apprehension or anxiety about coming to counselling to be present.

- The client can choose as few or as many of the prompt words or phrases that interest them most. They complete and extend these, either choosing the most interesting or working through the whole sheet, completing and extending all prompts.
- Let the client know there is no need to worry about grammar, spelling or handwriting. They are encouraged to use language that is easiest for them. This could be their first language.
- Encourage spontaneity: Suggest the client try not to plan responses. Instead, invite them to observe the words and phrases that form in their mind as they read the prompt. Then go with the flow!
- Advise them to try not to limit or censor what they write. Assure them they can keep their written responses private – if they wish.
- Their writing does not need to make sense, or to have a link with what came before.
- If no words or phrases emerge, the client simply moves on to the next starter. If they wish, they can return later to any missed ones or can choose to ignore them.
- When the client feels finished, they are invited to take some time to review their writing.

Activity 4.2 Sentence Starter Worksheet: *About Coming to Counselling*

- *Read through these sentence starters and complete the sentences in any way that pops into your mind. You don't need to worry about spelling or grammar or handwriting!! You may choose to draw your response, or prefer to choose objects from the collection that seem to fit with your words and thoughts.*
- *You can decide later if you want to share what you have written with the counsellor. You can keep what you have written private or talk about it – it's your choice.*
- I'm here because …
- What I don't want is …
- I'd rather be …
- My friends/parents/teachers think I'm …
- The main problem is …
- What I want is …
- *Can you take a moment to read through what you wrote?*
- *Can you underline any words that seem most important?*
- *What is the most interesting sentence?*
- *Is there a sentence you would be willing to share with the counsellor?*

Activity 4.3 Conversation Starters for Adolescents: *My Thoughts about Me*

- I think everything would be better if …
- The things I don't like are …
- What I need to say is …
- I worry about …
- I feel alone when …
- People tell me I should …
- If I could change anything it would be …
- What I really want is …

Activity 4.4 Reflection and Conversation Starters: *At the End of a Session*

- What I liked best was …
- The most difficult thing was …
- I felt good when …
- I was upset by …
- The strongest feeling was …
- One new idea is …
- I would like to know more about …

Activity 4.5 Reflection and Conversation Starters: *Who Am I?*

- In the past I used to …
- I now often feel …
- Inside my body I feel …
- I need to say …
- What worries me most …
- Nobody knows …
- All my life …
- The things I love …
- In the future …

Activity 4.6 Reflection and Conversation Starters: *More about Me*

- I often feel …
- I most regret …
- Other people …
- I am best when …
- What bothers me lately is …
- The happiest time …
- My parents …
- What I most want to change is …
- I need more …
- I wish …

Activity 4.7 Reflection and Conversation Starters: *The Voices of Others in My Life*

- People often tell me …
- Friends say to me …
- My family …
- When I was younger …
- What I've learned …
- My teachers say …
- My heroes are …

Activity 4.8 Reflection and Conversation Starters: *Thinking about the Future*

- The most important thing …
- My dream is …
- I am excited by …
- What I love in nature …
- My perfect day …
- I will feel happier …

- My safe place …
- My next challenges are …
- I want to make …
- I believe the future will be …

Review and Reflection Guidelines

Look over what you have written. Does anything stand out for you?

- *Can you underline or highlight words that seem most important.*
- *Which response is the most interesting to you?*
- *Could you extend these with some more writing?*
- *Are any statements or words contradictory?*

Take a few minutes to write or talk about how you feel after completing the writing and reflection.

- Invite the client to identify what on the page is most important for them.

Variations: If writing is not the client's preferred medium:

- try the activity as a verbal discussion
- respond to starters with a cartoon, or abstract colours and lines
- select miniatures for each starter.

Activity 4.9 Journaling Focus: *Reviewing Counselling So Far*

Suggested Age Range: 12–19 years
Materials: pen, paper

These questions can be used after a series of counselling sessions to provide focus for client self-understanding through journaling at home. They could also be offered as a means for the counsellor to obtain feedback.

Instructions

Write a response to each of these in your journal. Write as much or as little as you like:

1. *Focus inside yourself for a moment. Is there any struggle with what you have learnt through counselling?*
2. *Which session activities would you like to work with more?*
3. *Was there an activity that most helped you to feel free to be yourself? Was there one that was not helpful?*
4. *Note how your energy levels have been lately. Have you noticed anything about the ups and downs of your energy?*

5. *Do you have any new ideas or hopes about your future direction?*
6. *Are there any feelings, thoughts or memories you still want to talk about?*

Re-read what you have written. Are there any responses you would discuss with your counsellor in the next session?

Activity 4.10 Positive Writing: ***Gratitude and Joy Resource***

Suggested Age Range: From 12 years

Materials: Pen, *Gratitude & Joy Resource Worksheet* and crayons or coloured pencils

Aim: This activity from the field of positive psychology aims to reconnect the client with and record moments of joy and gratitude as a resource for wellbeing.

Reflection:
Relax as much as possible right now. Take a few deep breaths, and tune in to yourself.

Take a moment to recall:

- *Any people in your life you are grateful for, who add joy.*
- *A place in the world that evoked surprise and wonder.*
- *A time and place that evoked joy.*

Is there one of these that you would most like to focus on?

Take time now to let yourself recall as much as you can.

See if it is possible to recall:

- Other people who were involved
- The scenery, sights and sounds around you
- The way you felt in your body
- Colours, lines or shapes or images that best represent your recollection.

Take a moment to use the crayons to express on paper what you have recalled.

Extend these sentence starters:

- *When I feel joyful I …*
- *I am most grateful for …*
- *Recalling this could be most helpful when …*

Take some time to write what is most important for you from this recollection.

Worksheet: Gratitude and Joy Resource

The area I most wanted to recall and focus on:

Other people who were involved:

The scenery, sights and sounds around:

The way I felt in my body:

Colours, lines or shapes or images that best represent my recollection:

Words that sum up the experience:

Extend these sentence starters:

When I feel joyful I …

I am most grateful for …

Recalling this could be most helpful when …

What is most important for me from this activity:

Activity 4.11 Autobiography Plan: *The Chapters of My Life*

Suggested Age Range: From 14 years

Recognising and recounting our story is important for creating coherent episodes from the challenges of life. This helps re establish a sense of identity as well as gain some control over feelings of helplessness. This activity opens the door to knowing and appreciating ourselves more deeply.

- Write the *title* of your autobiography here (this can be delayed until chapter headings become apparent):
- Write out a minimum of seven *Life Chapter Titles* that represent significant life stages and events:

ONE:

TWO:

THREE:

FOUR:

FIVE:

SIX:

SEVEN:

INTO THE FUTURE:

- Then, for each chapter, *create one line* to describe the content and tone of the chapter.
- Last: Write the title of your final chapter – *Into the Future* – and a one-line description for it.

Activity 4.12 Therapeutic Use of Poetry Writing Activity: *Creating Acrostic Poems*

An acrostic is a poem in which the first letters of each line spell out a word or phrase. The word or phrase can be a name, a thing, a statement. Usually, the first letter of each line is capitalised. This makes it easier to see the word spelled out vertically down the page.

Acrostics are easy to write because they don't need to rhyme, and you don't need to worry about the rhythm of the lines. Each line can be as long or as short as you want it to be.

To create an acrostic:

1. Decide what to write about. For example: School or friends, happy times, worries.
2. Write your word down *vertically.*
3. Brainstorm words or phrases that describe your idea.
4. Place your brainstormed words or phrases on the lines that begin with the same letters.
5. Fill in the rest of the lines to create a poem.

The first step is to decide what you would like to write an acrostic poem about.

For this activity, try out using one of these as starters (see worksheet on the next page):

- *What I want*
- *My challenges*
- *Happiness is*

Writing Activity Worksheet: ***Creating Acrostic Poems***

W	
H	
A	
T	
I	
W	
A	
N	
T	

M	
Y	
C	
H	
A	
L	
E	
N	
G	
E	
S	

H	
A	
P	
P	
I	
N	
E	
S	
S	
I	
S	

Activity 4.13 Short Poems Help Focus: *Self-Reflective Haiku Writing*

Haiku – an unrhymed poetic form consisting of 17 syllables arranged in three lines of 5, 7 and 5 syllables respectively. The haiku first emerged in Japanese literature during the 17th century, as a terse reaction to elaborate poetic traditions, though it did not become known by the name *haiku* until the 19th century. Today the term *haiku* is used to describe all poems that use the three-line 17-syllable structure.

Based on a traditional Japanese poetic form, there are different ways to write haiku. The traditional pattern in English is to write the first and last of three lines with five syllables each, and the middle line with seven syllables. In other words, the pattern of syllables looks like this:

Line 1: 5 syllables
Line 2: 7 syllables
Line 3: 5 syllables

Another way to visualise the same thing:

1 2 3 4 5
1 2 3 4 5 6 7
1 2 3 4 5

Winter is coming.
Snow will be arriving soon.
We should rake the leaves.

1. Decide what aspect of yourself you are going to write about.
2. Think about what is different about your last line (think of it as your "punch line"). What observation do you want to make?
3. Start writing.
4. Don't forget to *count the syllables* as you read to make sure you've got the right pattern.
5. Finally, "centre" your poem on the page like the poems in this lesson.

Stargazing, I sense
the enduring universe
and my mortal self.
Bartholomew Williams

References

Altay, N., Kilicarslan-Toruner, E., & Sari, C. (2017). The effect of drawing and writing technique on the anxiety level of children undergoing cancer treatment. *European Journal of Oncology Nursing*, *28*, 1–6.

Baikie, K. A, Geerligs, L., & Wilhelm, K. (2012). Expressive writing and positive writing for participants with mood disorders: An online randomized controlled trial. *Journal of Affective Disorders*, *136*, 310–319.

Bohart, A. C., & Tallman, K. (1996). The active client: Therapy as self-help. *Journal of Humanistic Psychology*, *36*(3), 7–30.

Bolton, G., & Ihanus, J. (2011). Conversation about poetry/writing therapy: Two European perspectives. *Journal of Poetry Therapy*, *24*(3), 167–186.

Burton, C. M., & King, L. A. (2004). The health benefits of writing about intensely positive experiences. *Journal of Research in Personality*, *38*, 150–163.

Case, C., & Dalley, T. (1992). *The handbook of art therapy*. Tavistock/Routledge.

Connolly Baker, K., & Mazza, N. (2004). The healing power of writing: Applying the expressive/creative component of poetry therapy. *Journal of Poetry Therapy*, *17*(3), 141–154.

Combs, G., & Freedman, J. (1990). *Symbol, story and ceremony – Using metaphor in individual and family therapy*. W.W. Norton and Co.

Dalley, T., Rifkind, G., & Terry, K. (1993). *Three voices of art therapy: Image, client, therapist*. Routledge.

Deveney, C., & Lawson, P. (2022). Writing your way to well-being: An IPA analysis of the therapeutic effects of creative writing on mental health and the processing of emotional difficulties. *Counselling & Psychotherapy Research*, *22*, 292–300.

Diana, E., Khaerani, F. A., Khotimah, K., Wijaya, M. Z., & Purwaningrum, R. (2024). Using poetry as a counseling media to overcome adolescent problems: Systematic literature review. *Konseling Edukasi: Journal of Guidance and Counseling*, *7*(2), 251–266.

Edgar, K. (1979). A case of poetry therapy. *Psychotherapy: Theory, Research & Practice*, *16*(1), 104–106.

Freeman, D. C. (1997). Cognitive metaphor and literary theory: Towards the new philology. In *Deseret Language and Linguistic Society Symposium*, *23*(1), Article 5.

Freud, S. (1920). *Introductory lectures on psycho-analysis*. Freudian Association. https://freudianassociation.org/en/wp-content/uploads/Sigmund_Freud_1920_Introductory.pdf

Gardner, H. (1983). *Frames of mind: Theory of multiple intelligences*. Heinermann.

Greenbaum, C. A., & Javdani, S. (2017). Expressive writing intervention promotes resilience among juvenile justice-involved youth. *Children and Youth Services Review*, *73*, 220–229.

Haertl, K. L., & Ero-Phillips, A. M. (2019). The healing properties of writing for persons with mental health conditions. *Arts & Health*, *11*(1), 15–25.

Heimes, S. (2011). State of poetry therapy research. *The Arts in Psychotherapy*, *38*(1), 1–8.

Hoult, L. M., Wetherell, M. A., Edginton, T., & Smith, M. A. (2025). Positive expressive writing interventions, subjective health and wellbeing in non-clinical populations: A systematic review. *PLoS One*, *20*(5), e0308928.

Kenardy, J., & Piercy, J., A. (2006). Effect of information provision on trauma symptoms following therapeutic writing. *Australian Psychologist*, *41*(3), 205–218.

Kloser, K. (2013). Positive youth development through the use of poetry therapy: The contributing effects of language arts in mental health counseling with middle school-age children. *Journal of Poetry Therapy, 26*(4), 237–253.

Koppman, M. (2001). On the edge of life: Poetry helps cancer patients cope. *Annals of Long-Term Care, 9*(2), 68–72.

Landgarten, H. B. (1981). *Clinical art therapy: A comprehensive guide.* Brunner/Mazel.

Lusebrink, V. B. (1990). Levels of expression and systems approach to therapy. In V. B. Lusebrink (Ed.), *Imagery and visual expression in therapy* (pp. 91–114). Springer.

Lyddon, W. J., Clay, A. L., & Sparks, C. L. (2001). Metaphor and change in counseling. *Journal of Counseling & Development, 79*(3), 269–274.

MacCurdy, M. M. (2000). From trauma to writing. A theoretical model for practical use. In C. M. Anderson & M. M. MacCurdy (Eds.), *Writing and healing. Toward an informed practice* (pp. 158–200). National Council of Teachers of English.

Marano, G., Kotzalidis, G. D., Lisci, F. M., Anesini, M. B., Rossi, S., Barbonetti, S., & Mazza, M. (2025). The neuroscience behind writing: Handwriting vs. typing – Who wins the battle? *Life, 15*(3), 345.

McCulliss, D. (2011). Poetry Therapy. In L. L'Abate & L. G. Sweeney (Eds.), *Research on writing approaches in mental health: Studies in writing* (Vol. 3, pp. 93–114). Emerald Group.

Mugerwa, S., & Holden, J. D. (2012). Writing therapy: A new tool for general practice? *British Journal of General Practice, 62*(605), 661–663.

Oaklander, V. (1978). *Windows to our children. A Gestalt Therapy approach to children and adolescents.* Real People Press.

O'Brien, P., & Burnett, P. (2000). Counselling children using a multiple intelligences framework. *British Journal of Guidance and Counselling, 28*(3), 353–371.

Oster, G., & Gould, P. (1987). *Using drawings in assessment and therapy: A guide for mental health professionals.* Brunner/Mazel Inc.

Pardeck, J. T., & Markward, M. J. (1995). Bibliotherapy: Using books to help children deal with problems. *Early Child Development and Care, 106*, 75–90.

Payne, M. (2006). *Narrative therapy: An introduction for counsellors.* Sage.

Pearson, M., & Wilson, H. (2009). *Using expressive arts to work with mind, body and emotions. Theory and practice.* Jessica Kingsley Publishers.

Pennebaker, J. W., & Beall, S. K. (1986). Confronting a traumatic event. Toward an understanding of inhibition and disease. *Journal of Abnormal Psychology, 95*(3), 274–281.

Pennebaker, J. W., & Seagal, J. D. (1999). Forming a story: The health benefits of narrative. *Journal of Clinical Psychology, 55*, 1243–1254.

Peterkin, A. D., & Prettyman, A. A. (2009). Finding a voice: Revisiting the history of therapeutic writing. *Medical Humanities, 35*(2), 80–88.

Progoff, I. (1992). *At a journal workshop: Writing to access the power of the unconscious and evoke creative ability.* Penguin.

Raingruber, B. (2004). Using poetry to discover and share significant meanings in child and adolescent mental health nursing. *Journal of Child and Adolescent Psychiatric Nursing, 17*(1), 13–20.

Riordan, R. J. (1996). Scriptotherapy: Therapeutic writing as a counseling adjunct. *Journal of Counseling and Development, 74*, 263–269.

Ross, C. A. (2017). The benefits of therapeutic writing in acute psychiatric units. *Mental Health Practice, 20*(7), 33–38.

Round, E. K., Wetherell, M. A., Elsey, V., & Smith, M. A. (2022). Positive expressive writing as a tool for alleviating burnout and enhancing wellbeing in teachers and other full-time workers. *Cogent Psychology*, *9*(1), 2060628.

Rubin, J. A. (1978). *Child art therapy.* Van Norstrand Reinhold.

Ruini, C., & Mortara, C. C. (2022). Writing technique across psychotherapies – From traditional expressive writing to new positive psychology interventions: A narrative review. *Journal of Contemporary Psychotherapy*, *52*, 23–34.

Shahrabady, S., Gholami, S., Afsharloo, S., Fakhreazizi, S., Izadi, M., & Hojjati, H. (2021). The effect of poetry reading on self-concept of primary adolescents. *International Journal of Adolescent Medicine and Health*, *33*(6), 457–461.

Van der Oord, S., Lucassen, S., Van Emmerik, A. A. P., & Emmelkamp, P. M. (2010). Treatment of post-traumatic stress disorder in children using cognitive behavioural writing therapy. *Clinical Psychology & Psychotherapy: An International Journal of Theory & Practice*, *17*(3), 240–249.

Waters, T. (2002). The therapeutic use of story writing: Can literacy work provide a therapeutic context in which to support children with emotional and behavioural difficulties in mainstream schools? *Psychodynamic Practice*, *8*, 343–358.

Wright, J., & Chung, M. C. (2001). Mastery or mystery? Therapeutic writing: A review of the literature. *British Journal of Guidance and Counselling*, *29*(3), 277–291.

5 Sounds, Songs and Rhythms

Music in Counselling

Using Music Therapeutically

Since ancient times, music has been used to enhance wellbeing and reduce pain and suffering (Kemper & Danhauer, 2005). Listening to music stimulates the brain and the body–mind connection; it can reactivate speech centres of the brain, prompt memory and improve gait and coordination (Brey, 2006). Music can create and alter moods, facilitate the expression of emotions and reduce stress and anxiety. It can be used to capture and focus attention, elicit memories, communicate feelings and create a sense of community (Mandsager, Newsome & Glass, 1997).

In recommending the use of music in counselling, we are sensitive to and somewhat awed by the vast arena of Music Therapy skills, knowledge and research. Qualified music therapists have postgraduate training and also have music performance training in their backgrounds. We do not confuse the use of music in ET or in counselling generally with Music Therapy. Some of the receptive Music Therapy methods can, however, be safely used by counsellors.

The profession of Music Therapy began to develop in the USA during WW I and WW II, when music was used in Veterans Administration Hospitals as an intervention to address mood in relation to traumatic war injuries. In 1950 a professional organisation was formed by a collaboration of music therapists that worked with veterans, "mentally retarded", hearing/visually impaired and psychiatric populations. This was the birth of the USA National Association for Music Therapy. The Australian Music Therapy Association (AMTA) was formed in 1975, and publishes the *Australian Journal of Music Therapy.*

How does music therapy work? Within the therapeutic relationship, the music therapist uses the specific elements of music to elicit emotional, physiological, psychological and social and spiritual responses from their clients, in order to support restoration and improvement of health, functioning and wellbeing (AMTA, n.d.).

Basic methods used in traditional Music Therapy include improvisation where the client and/or therapist may spontaneously create music. Re-creative experiences where pre-composed music is used include performing and interpreting. Composition experiences, where the therapist and/or client create a

DOI: 10.4324/9781003671879-5

specific enduring musical product, such as writing songs, lyrics or instrumental pieces, as well as creating audio or video projects.

The role of music in the therapeutic process can include music as a regulating force in therapy, sometimes with listening and sometimes with music-making at the forefront. In everyday life, people regularly use music for regulating their emotions (Skånland, 2013). Music as a regulating force has been found to be efficient with adolescents (Saarikallio & Erkkila, 2007).

Receptive experiences of music are the ones most safely incorporated into ET. For example, a client listens to recorded music and charts their responses, sharing thoughts, feelings or imagery, either verbally or through drawing, use of clay, or painting. Sampling and selecting preferred music as a collaborative process with the counsellor can act as a bonding and communication activity early in therapy.

Some of the ET music activities draw on The Bonny Method (Bonny & Savary, 1973), a Guided Imagery and Music programme developed by Helen Bonny (1921–2010). The process typically saw a therapist first involve a client or group in a period of progressive relaxation, explaining that soon they would hear recorded background music. After being guided to focus on "travelling inwardly" and listening attentively to the music tracks, participants would be invited to share their imagery experiences. Sharing times related to what was "witnessed" or evoked while listening to the music. This provided a medium for exploring implicit memory, forgotten issues and/or experiences that may be too painful to discuss directly.

Research shows that listening to live or recorded music can be useful for relaxation, reducing stress, reducing anxiety and depression, managing pain, regulating body functions (e.g., heart rate, breathing), generating imagery and accessing the sub-conscious (Bailes, 2003). Listening to classical music is known to evoke strong emotions, including feelings of pleasure (Krumhansl, 1997).

Research findings indicate that the use of music in therapy with children and adolescents can be highly beneficial (Gold et al., 2004). Most benefits of using music in therapy with young clients result from improvisation and verbal reflection (Gold et al., 2007).

Music is often used in ET to help a client develop emotional literacy. Emotional literacy includes: The ability to sense and locate emotions in the body, being able to recognise emotions, name them, communicate about them and speculate about causes. Ability with emotional literacy assists the process of therapy, offering support for integration of emotional experiences, therapeutic release and in developing emotional regulation and enhancing communication about emotion. (See more in Chapter 7).

Use of music will particularly suit clients whose preference is a musical/rhythmic intelligence (Gardner, 2006). Gardner's musical intelligence involves skill in performance, composition and appreciation of musical patterns. It encompasses the capacity to recognise and compose musical pitches, tones and rhythms (Smith, 2008).

Early estimates suggested that approximately 4% of the population experience tone deafness (Cox, 1947; Joyner, 1968), and the term amusia is generally applied to individuals whose processing of one or more aspects of music indicates a shortfall (Levitin & Tirovolas, 2009). This can alert us to increase sensitivity to any times when inviting engagement with music may not be welcomed or responded to in a way that proves useful.

Using Recorded Music

When using recorded music, consider how to choose appropriate tracks. It is best to choose longer tracks (i.e., over three minutes), with a consistency in mood, volume and speed. Music can be used simply to provide privacy, as an energetic background to encourage expression, or conversely as a holding space for quiet time and for relaxation.

Avoid music with words in a language known to your client. While clients may like to bring in songs that are meaningful to them for discussion, if we offer music with words it could prescribe a focus rather than allow spontaneous responses. Frightening music (e.g., horror movie soundtracks with abrupt and disjointed sounds) is also avoided. Music that is too familiar, or classical Western or some Eastern music, that usually is not fully appreciated by young clients would also be chosen with great care. If possible, it is good to avoid using music that has been ultra-condensed in the recording process.

Take time to become familiar with music equipment. When changing, starting, or stopping music, turn the volume up and down to avoid audio shocks. Consider if you want a helpful consistent rhythm or music with almost no regular beats. Check the melody: is it in the foreground or background? Is it too intrusive, attractive, or overly emotional?

Playing with Music and Sound Activities

As a rapport-building activity, allow the client to listen to some of your music and discuss their responses. Invite them to bring some of their favourite music to the session, listen to it and discuss. Acknowledge similarities and differences in your likes and dislikes.

Spending time exploring percussion and drums can support expression, communication and stress release. When you have access to a keyboard, representational sounds, spontaneous or improvisational songs, depiction of a person, place or experience and expressions of a mood can all be evoked. Of course, for clients who clearly have an affinity with music, playing and composing something at home can bring mood-enhancing benefits from creative expression.

MUSIC ACTIVITIES

Activity 5.1 Improvising: *Keyboard Rhythms*

Aim: For "joining" with the client, creating a bond and encouraging their expression. No musical ability is required.

Materials: A keyboard, e.g., piano, small electronic keyboard. If no keyboard is available, explore downloading a keyboard onto your iPad.

The client sits at the keyboard, is invited to take a moment to tune in to self, take a few deep breaths, then have some fun with their expression. Invite them to express:

- some sounds from their life, e.g., what the winds sound like; what it sounds like in the playground at school, etc.
- spontaneous, improvisational songs
- depict a few significant people, places or experiences
- express a mood, feeling, or event
- some tunes or songs they may have learnt at home.

Activity 5.2 Emotional Expression Activity: *Talking Drums Using Rhythm and Percussion*

Suggested Age Range: From seven years

Materials: Drums and percussion instruments, drawing materials, A3 size drawing paper divided into four segments.

- Warm-up: Explore the sound of the drum
  - *How much noise can you make?*
  - Drum along with pre-recorded drumming music,
  - Interact with client – set a rhythm, the client follows, then swap roles.
- Client is invited to move about while playing the instruments.
- Client is invited to play and create rhythms and sounds that go with and express the feelings of to these experiences:
  1. *A happy time, a happy place*
  2. *A not-so-happy time, a sad time*
  3. *The three or four most important people in their life* (respond to each separately)
  4. *A time of anger, or being at a place they didn't like*
  5. *The most peaceful or enjoyable time, or activity*

After each expression:

- Ask the client if there is anything they would like to say

- Invite them to quickly put colours and lines in the segments to show how it felt.

• Client is invited to see if there are a few lines of a song or a few words that go with the sounds they are making.

Integration

- After the last round, invite the client to tune in to self for a moment, then draw in a circle:
  - How they feel inside with colours and lines
  - Add a few words that go with the feelings
  - And then share the final mood
- Final stage: Invite the client to tune in to self again and see if they would want to drum and express how they feel now, and/or express with drumming what they "see" in their integration drawing.

Activity 5.3 Generating Interaction: *Yes, No, I Would Rather*

Materials: A3 paper (folded into four segments), crayons, pen. Recorded music: four tracks

Aims: A quick activity to generate client interest in using music in the session, through providing freedom to express likes and dislikes to music you choose.

Select *four* very different tracks and play them – alternate between tracks you hope the client will like and ones you suspect they may not like.

- Client numbers the segments on the page: 1, 2, 3, 4.
- Play tracks, one at a time.
- Client listens and responds:
  - By writing *"Yes"*, *"No"* or "*I would rather …*" in the segment
  - Adds some colours and lines to show their response.
- Discuss their responses, with a focus on any alternatives they suggest.
- Invite the client to bring – or find on iTunes, YouTube, Spotify, etc. – music they enjoy, and share and discuss this with you.

Activity 5.4 Generating Interaction: *Remembering Feelings*

Materials: A3 paper, crayons, two tracks of music

Aims: To support a client to open to internal experience and emotional memory.

Select *two tracks of music* that express very different moods. (e.g., sadness and happiness)

- Client stands, takes a few deep breaths, closes eyes and opens ears.
- Say: **Listen to the music**:
    - *Can you feel what happens inside you as you listen?*
    - *Is there a way it affects your mood or seems to have a mood of its own?*
    - *Are there any memories or pictures that the music brings to your mind?*
    - *Any times when you have felt like this music?*
- *Could you* draw quickly *now? See if you could express whatever lines, colours, shapes, images you feel go with the music. Don't think much about it, let it happen.*
- *Would you be able to* add a word *or two that go with the moods or memories.*
- Repeat with second track.
- **Discuss**: *Would you be willing to share what you have drawn?*
    - *Was it easy or hard to do?*
    - *Have you ever felt similar to any of these tracks?*
    - *Did the music remind you of anything in your life?*

Activity 5.5 Body Awareness: *Responding to Rhythm*

Materials: A3 paper, crayons. Select three music tracks with clear, repeated and different rhythms.

Aims: To explore movement responses to rhythms in order to integrate body awareness and spontaneity, for supporting client engagement, reflection, communication, relaxation and wellbeing.

Client stands. Listens to and responds to one track at a time.

Instructions

- *Stretch, breathe and shake for a moment.*
- *Tune in to your body.*
- *As you listen to the track:*
    - *See if you can "see" in your mind's eye the types of lines the rhythm suggests, and quickly express these on the paper.*
    - *Tune into the music again, and see if you can notice any responses to the music in your body.*
    - *Are there any parts of your body that feel they would like to move in response to the music? Try out some movements.*
    - *Which movements feel right to you? See if you could repeat these and bring them into a sequence, a bit like a short dance.*
    - *Could you show this movement to me (or others in a group setting), and I will try to copy you.*
- *What words could you put with it? Could you write these on the page beside the lines?*
- *Would you like to make up a name for this movement, for your dance?*

Repeat for the three tracks.

Integration

After three tracks, invite the client to rest and reflect on:

- Their own natural or preferred rhythms, i.e., what comes most naturally?
- Places, people, events that evoke different internal speeds or rhythms.
- Times when different rhythms would be most useful.

Activity 5.6 Creating Rhythm Metaphors: *Expressing Feelings*

Materials: Drums, percussion instruments, drawing materials, A3 paper.

Aim: To provide non-verbal ways to contact and express feelings through sounds and rhythms.

1. Tune in to yourself.

2. Warm-up:
Explore the sound of the drum and instruments:

- *How much noise can you make?*
- Explore differences using left and right hands on the drum.
- Interact with client – set a rhythm, the client follows, then swap roles.
- Drum along with pre-recorded drumming music.

3. Client is invited to *play and create rhythms* and sounds that go with and express the feelings of to these experiences in a new "drum language".

- *A happy time, a happy place.*
- *A troublesome person in their life.*
- *A time of anger or frustration, or being at a place they really didn't like, or with people they didn't like.*
- *The most peaceful or enjoyable time, activity or place.*

4. Tune in again.
5. Client is invited to *draw* how they feel now and see if there are a *few words* that go with this.

Integration:

6. Discuss:

- *What did you notice about using the drum and the instruments?*
- *How do you feel now?*

- *Any differences between how they felt at the start and when they tuned in again in Step 4?*

Activity 5.7 Responding to Music with Art: *Drawing the Music*

Suggested Age Range: 8 to 18 years

Materials: Drawing materials: Crayons and A3 Worksheet (Fig 5.1) or plain paper

Preparation: Select three music tracks that express different feelings and energies and moods: e.g., strong drumming, gentle flowing music, happy playful music, dance rhythms.

Choose music without words.

Instructions

The client is invited to stand and take a couple of slow, full breaths.
Play the first track of music (for approximately 1–2 minutes – fairly loud).
Invite careful listening. Ask:

- *What mood goes with this music?*
- *Is there anywhere you can feel the music inside you?*
- *Does the music make you want to move?*
- *Does your body say YES or NO to the music?*
- *Is there a colour that goes with this music?*
- *Is there a shape or some lines or pictures that go with this music?*

Turn the music down a little and repeat the track while they draw. Students are now invited to:

- *Draw quickly now in the circle – use whatever lines, colours, shapes, pictures you feel go with the music.*
- *Add a word or two – on the lines under the circle – that goes with the way the music makes you feel.*

Repeat the drawing step with each selection of music.

Integration

Clients are invited to show their drawings and share what is most interesting to them.

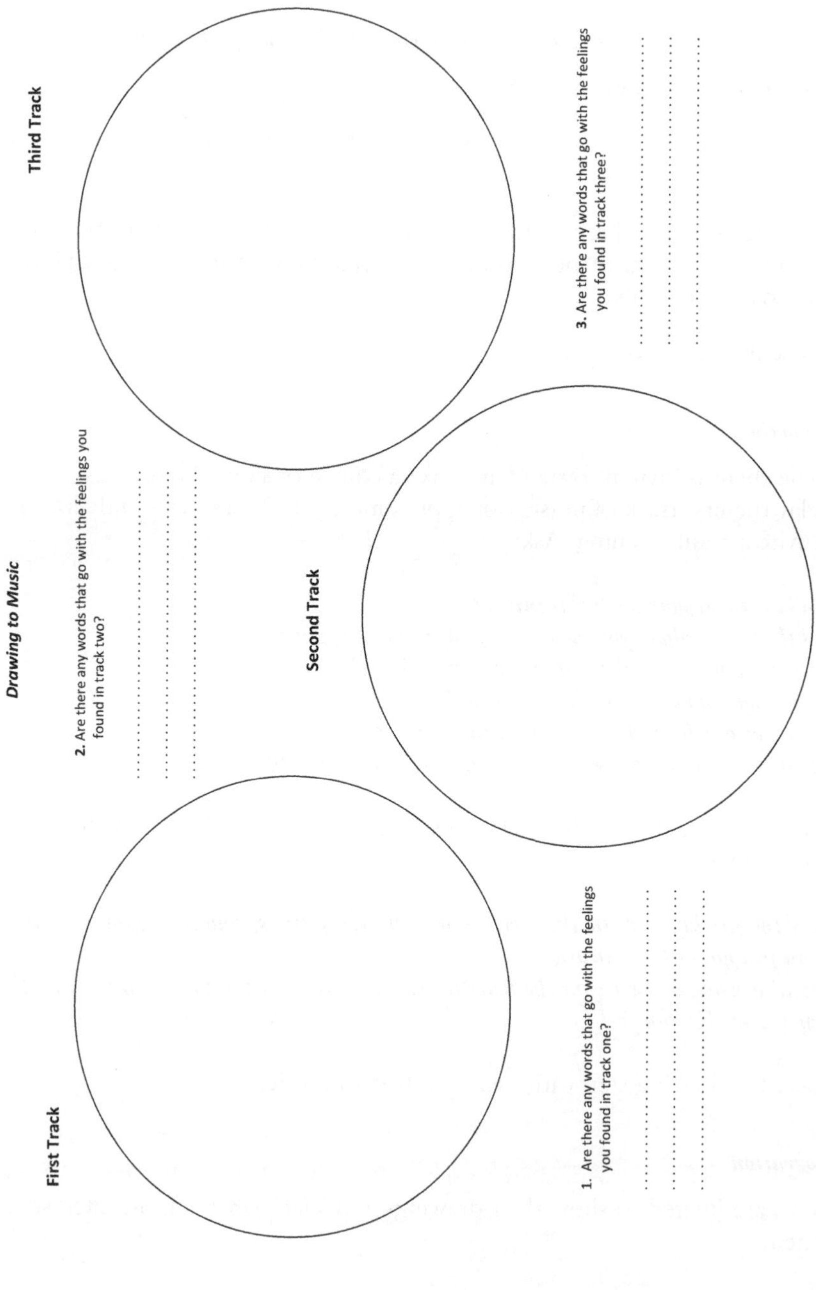

Figure 5.1 Worksheet – drawing to music.

They are invited to talk about:

- any tracks they particularly liked or disliked
- how they felt in response to the music
- whether the music reminded them of anything in their life
- any times when they felt like any of the tracks.

Music Suggestions

1. *Last of the Mohicans* – Trevor Jones – Film soundtrack – Track 8
2. *Titania – Mike Rowland* – Track 1
3. *Culture* – Chris Spheeris – track 8 (1.00–5.16)

Activity 5.8 Emotional Literacy Worksheet: *Finding Feelings in Music*

Age Range: From approximately nine years

Materials: Worksheet – *Finding Feelings in Music* (Fig 5.2); music player, four tracks of different types of music that have clear emotional tones; crayons, pen, Feeling Word List (Appendix, p. 252).

Aim: Opens conversation, deepens dialogue. Can help the counsellor observe the client's preferred intelligence. An introduction to more specific self-discovery.

Instructions

- Initiate a *brief conversation about music*, the types of music both client and counsellor like.
- Explain that the worksheet is designed to help us learn more about feelings and how to talk about them.
- Review columns on the worksheet and options for responding.
- Give client the option to share (or not to share) the responses they record on the worksheet.
- Support the client to relax and tune in to self, prior to playing tracks.

Process

- Invite client to listen to the sounds around them before the music starts, to "open the ears"
- Play first music track. The client listens, then fills in the columns in their preferred order. Repeat the track while the worksheet is being completed, if need be.
- Offer the *Feeling Word Lists* to support responses to the 5th column (see Appendix).

WORKSHEET: ***Finding Feelings in Music***

The Music Track	Colours, line and shapes in the music	This music makes me think of . . .	Feeling words that go with the music	Any times I have felt like this music
1				
2				
3				
4				

Figure 5.2 Worksheet – finding feelings in music.

- Between tracks invite the client to stretch, wriggle, move and re-focus within.
- Suggest taking a slow, full breath or two to help re-focus.

Consider if the client prefers to debrief each track before proceeding to the next. Complete responding to all four tracks.

Integration

- Invite the client to review the sheet and reflect on:
  - the response or column that came first
  - track they liked most, track they liked least
  - track that had the strongest impact
  - column that was easiest to complete/fill out
  - any parts of the worksheet that stand out, or attract their interest
  - discuss any feelings or memories evoked.
- With client's agreement, take time to discuss what has been written in the final column.
- The counsellor and client together may recognise particular responses that the client could explore further.

Music Suggestions for Finding Feelings in Music Worksheet Activity

Set 1

1. *Penny Whistle Song* Tr.#9 from soundtrack *The Power of One* – Hans Zimmer
2. Main theme from soundtrack – *Out of Africa* – John Barry – Track #1
3. Track #2 from soundtrack – *1492: Conquest of Paradise* – Vangelis
4. Track #1 from *The Secret Garden* – David Sun

Set 2

1. Track #3 from soundtrack *Gladiator* – Hans Zimmer
2. Track #1 from soundtrack *Braveheart* – James Horner
3. Track #3 from *All One Tribe* (Thunderdrums II) – Scot Fitzgerald
4. Track #1 from *Crystal Cascades* – Chris Buckman

Set 3

1. Track #7 from soundtrack *Dances with Wolves* – John Barry
2. Track #12 from soundtrack compilation *Moviola* – John Barry
3. Track #7 from *Guem – Percussion* – Guem
4. Track #1 from *Mariner* – Tony O'Connor

Choosing Recorded Music to Support Sessions

The selections of music listed here are suggestions only. All are available on compact disc. Many are available on streaming services. The tracks listed are in order of recommendation for a particular mood. Children and adolescents may have a preference for their own music. The client may like to share their music with you. Discuss preferences with the client.

Emotional Release Processing and for Bioenergetics

Serge Dow: *In Touch with Light*
Gabrielle Roth:
Initiation: Tracks 2, 3 and 6
Ritual from track 2 onwards
Waves, especially tracks 2 and 3
Totem especially tracks 3, 1, 2
Anugama: *Exotic Dance* especially track 1
(Nightingale Records NGH – CD – 311)
Brent Lewis: *Earth Tribe Rhythms – The Primitive Truth* esp. tracks 1, 6, 7
Scott Fitzgerald: *Thunderdrums I* especially tracks 7, 6, 5
Thunderdrums II – All One Tribe (celebration Tr. 3)
Guem: *Percussions* tracks 1, 7, 9, 3 are best (Le Chants du Monde)
James Asher: *Feet in the Soil* – especially trk 5 (New Earth Records – NE 9512 – 2)
Tigers of the Raj – especially trks 4, 1, 8, 9 (New Earth Records NE 9805 – 2)
Red Cosmic Earth: *Drums on Earth* – track 1 and others

Empowering/Heroic/Triumphant

Vangelis: From the film *1492*, especially tracks 2, 5, 6
Antarctica – track 1
Hans Zimmer: Soundtrack – *Gladiator* tracks 3, 9

Tenderness/Grief and Loss

John Barry: Soundtrack *Indecent Proposal* – track 7 (25 mins)
Mark Knopfler: Soundtrack *Princess Bride*
Ennio Morricone: Soundtrack *Love Affair,* especially tracks 5, 12, 11, 10, 6
James Horner: Quieter tracks from the film *Braveheart* tracks 1, 4, 16, 18, 7

Music to Support Grief and Anger Activities

The tracks listed are in order of our recommendation for the particular mood.

Grief, Sadness, Loss:
John Barry: Soundtrack *Out of Africa,* MCAD 6158
soundtrack *Dances With Wolves* tracks 2, 3, 8, 9, 12, 13;
compilation CD *Moviola,* especially tracks 13, 12, 6, 8, 5
Mike Rowland: *Titania* – all tracks
Mark Knopfler: Soundtrack *Last Exit to Brooklyn,* only tracks 4, 9, 1.
James Horner: Soundtrack *Legends of the Fall* tracks 6, 3, 9, 10, 12, 2
soundtrack *Braveheart* tracks 7, 2, 16, 11, 4
David Pickvance: *Tempest* – all tracks
Wyndham Hill: *In Search of Angels* – all tracks
Tony O'Connor: *Windseeker* – all tracks Studio Horizon HORCD40

Anger and Power:
Trevor Jones: Soundtrack *The Last of the Mohicans,* tracks 8, 5, 2, 1, 9
Jerry Goldsmith: Soundtrack *Total Recall,* tracks 1, 9, 3, 5
Gabrielle Roth: *Initiation,* track 2 and 3
Scott Fitzgerald: *Thunderdrums* – especially tracks 7, 6 and 5
Drummers of Burundi
Phillip Glass: Soundtrack *Powaqqatsi* especially track 7
James Horner: Soundtrack of *Braveheart* tracks 13, 5, 10, 14
Vangelis: Soundtrack *Antarctica* tracks 3, 1, 5.
soundtrack *1492,* especially tracks 2, 6, 5, 9;
compilation *Themes*
soundtrack *Blade Runner*
John Barry: Soundtrack *Dances With Wolves,* tracks 7, 15, 1, 10, 16
Serge Douw: *In Touch With Light* – all tracks

Integration and Background Music:
Phillip Chapman: *Keeper of Dreams* (New World NWCD 164)
Cary Lewincamp: *The Sky in your Eyes; Home; A Fresh Wind*
David Pickvance: *Tempest* (New World ELK 001)
Windham Hill Collection: *In Search of Angels*

Stillness, Relaxation, Letting-go:
Ennio Morricone: Soundtrack *City of Joy,* tracks 7, 2, 9, 15, 19, 10, 3
Terry Oldfield: *Cascade* all tracks (from New World Music NWC 140)
Illuminations (from New World Music)
Tony O'Connor: *Mariner,* all tracks
Jon Mark: *Alhambra,* most tracks
Anugama: *Spiritual Environment* Track 1 (Nightingale Records NGH-CD-319)
Simon Lewis: *Southern Mystique* tracks 1, and 7
David Lanz: *Christofori's Dream* all tracks
David Sun: *The Secret Garden* – all tracks (new World Music – NWC 205)
Healing Massage – New World Music (MBSCD 914)

Strong Movement and Celebration:
Sirocco: *Port of Call*, tracks 2, 3, 9, 8 (Jarra Hill Records – CD JHR 2009)
Wetland Suite (ABC Music) tracks 1, 3, 11, 12, 17
Chris Spheeris: *Culture* tracks 1, 2, 4 – also 3 (more gentle)
Hans Zimmer: *The Power of One* (ST) tracks 9, 12, 14

References

Australian Music Therapy Association (AMTA). (n.d.). https://www.austmta.org.au/

Bailes, F. (2003). *Experimental studies in musical imagery: Implicit and explicit cognition.* Proceedings of the 5th Triennial ESCOM Conference, Hanover University of Music and Drama.

Bonny, H. L., & Savary, L. M. (1973). *Music and your mind: Listening with a new consciousness.* Harper & Row.

Brey, R. L. (2006). Voices of the human spirit: Speaking out, singing out. *Neurology Now*, *2*(1), 5.

Cox, I. (1947). Tone deafness. *Music Educator's Journal*, *34*, 62–63.

Gardner, H. (2006). *The development and education of mind.* Taylor & Francis Limited.

Gold, C., Voracek, M., & Wigram, T. (2004). Effects of music therapy for children and adolescents with psychopathology: A meta-analysis. *Journal of Child Psychology and Psychiatry*, *45*(6), 1054–1063.

Gold, C., Wigram, T., & Voracek, M. (2007). Predictors of change in music therapy with children and adolescents: The role of therapeutic techniques. *Psychology and Psychotherapy: Theory, Research and Practice*, *80*(4), 577–589.

Joyner, D. R. (1968). The montone problem. *Journal of Research in Music Education*, *17*(1), 115–124.

Kemper, K. J., & Danhauer, S. C. (2005). Music as therapy. *Southern Medical Journal*, *98*(3), 282–287.

Krumhansl, C. L. (1997). An exploratory study of musical emotions and psychophysiology. *Canadian Journal of Experimental Psychology*, *51*, 336–353. https://doi.org/10.1037/1196-1961.51.4.336

Levitin, D. J., & Tirovolas, A. K. (2009). Current advances in the cognitive neuroscience of music. *Annals of the New York Academy of Sciences*, *1156*(1), 211–231.

Mandsager, N., Newsome, D., & Glass, S. (1997). Music as metaphor. In *Annual Conference of the North Carolina Counseling Association*, Greensboro, NC.

Saarikallio, S., & Erkkila, J. (2007). The role of music in adolescents' mood regulation. *Psychology of Music*, *35*(1), 88–109.

Skånland, M. S. (2013). Everyday music listening and affect regulation: The role of MP3 players. *International Journal of Qualitative Studies on Health and Well-being*, *8*(1), 20595. https://doi.org/10.3402/qhw.v8i0.20595

Smith, T. M. (2008). *Integrating multiple intelligences and andragogical principles into a preservice teacher education program.* Walden University.

6 Muscles, Bone and Skin

Somatic Awareness, Movement and Relaxation

Introduction to Somatics

At the core of an ET approach to including somatic awareness in counselling and therapy is an understanding of the uniqueness of each client and the relationship they have with their physical self. Incorporating focused attention to the body in counselling and therapy has developed from a number of approaches: Body-oriented Therapy, Somatic Therapy, Somatic experiencing, Sensorimotor Psychotherapy, Bioenergetic Analysis, as well as traditions such as Yoga and Tai Chi. Bodywork, as outlined in other approaches, is a specific technique not used in the same way in ET, particularly with young clients.

This chapter provides some distinctive ideas and structured activities for enhancing somatic awareness through

- body focus processes
- creating tension and movement in the body to reduce stress
- exploring expression through movement
- using movement as preparation for relaxation and stillness
- body posture activities for improving wellbeing.

Why enhance body awareness? Intentional connection with the body as a "whole", developing an ability to recognise body sensations and cues, as well as integration of mind and body processing are activities designed to foster a positive relationship for a client with their body. The benefit of a revised or re-visioned relationship with the body can be found in the experience of the body as more than a structure that can carry out physical tasks or, conversely, has betrayed the individual through body discomfort, illness or pain. Rather than regarding disparate aspects of the body as purely a useful mechanical resource, a person can come to understand how they may have unconsciously taken their body for granted, and how a "split" from body awareness contributes to feelings of dysregulation, disintegration and disembodiment (Gyllensten et al., 2010, 2019; Mehling et al., 2011).

Body sensations have been found to have an impact on wellbeing and health (Gyllensten et al., 2010). Body sensations cue awareness of emotion, underlie emotions, form the basis for weighing consequences, deciding direction

DOI: 10.4324/9781003671879-6

and identifying preferences (Damasio, 2003), as well as reducing tendencies for impulsivity in reacting to others. Awareness of body signals establishes a foundation for accessing somatically based emotional messages that moderate reconnection with a more emotionally balanced state.

Somatic awareness – *through stillness, focusing,* can lead to
↓
Emotional awareness
↓
which makes more possible
↓
Cognitive awareness
↓
and
↓
Awareness of behaviour
↓
Which can lead to
↓
Informed Choice

Body ownership, a term used by Tsakiris et al. in their 2007 study of agency and body ownership, relates, in part, to awareness of bodily experiences such as touch. From an ET perspective, body ownership has significance for counselling with younger clients as an important support for their sense of personal agency. A healthy sense of personal agency can assist in the transition from dependence to independence for adolescents. In younger children (and adolescents), understanding body ownership can positively mediate comfort seeking, pursuit of affection and developing emotional connection with self and others. The kind of relationships young children and adolescents establish with their peers, and most importantly with themselves, means that body awareness becomes an integral part of counselling support for connecting mental and body experiences. Help for a young person to extend their ability to recognise and creatively represent information originating from the body may mitigate susceptibility to a negative self-concept and unproductive and unhealthy interpersonal relating.

Let's look now at one way ET suggests we can offer integration of mind and body. The first activity – "Does your nose say no?" is offered as preparation prior to more focused attention on signals from the body. At first, a young client may not feel safe or comfortable to engage in an experiential activity such as *What my body tells* me (see p. 139). From a counsellor's assessment of the client's bodily state, it may be advisable for there to be a slower, steadier entry into talking with the counsellor about body and body sensations. "Does your nose say no?" gives a client an opportunity to experience a sense of control about the pacing and content of the therapy session. They can say no! They can say yes! It's their choice.

Activity 6.1 Preparation for Body Focus: *Does Your Nose Say No?*

Materials*:* Prepared body outline shape (A3 size), crayons, pencil.

Aim: To support recovery from dissociation, by inviting a client to explore readiness for somatic focus, to begin to reconnect with somatic experience. The activity provides a process by which a client can gradually begin to listen and recognise messages from body symptoms. Another aim of this activity is to establish a way for the client to practise having choice in the activity and then, hopefully, become interested to proceed in risking a return to somatic awareness, at their own rate of readiness.

Client has body outline and crayons beside them. They are invited to get comfortable, leaning back on cushions, or reclining on a floor rug or carpet.

The counsellor gives an overview of the activity and checks if the client has understood and, importantly, is willing to proceed.

> *Counsellor: The aim of this activity is to ask different parts of your body if they would be willing to join in with the activity. To see if they would be OK for you to focus on how that parts feels today. It may seem a bit strange at first, but we are simply going to ask each part of your body if they are willing or ready to get involved, and see if it has anything to say. Did you know it is possible for each part to have an opinion? Each part can say "Yes", "No", or "Maybe" or anything else it wants to say. Or it may not want to answer. Would that be OK with you?*
>
> *OK, let's start with your nose. Take a moment to focus on your nose. Let's ask it if it would be willing to play this game and be the centre of attention for a few moments.*

Allow time for a response.

The client is invited to write the response from their nose on the body outline.

The next step is to ask each of the extremities if they would be willing to participate: E.g., feet and toes, hands and fingers, ears, etc. If the client remains comfortable, invite them to focus closer to the centre of the body: E.g., arms, legs, head. Finally, if the client remains at ease and engaged, take the focus to more "vulnerable" parts of the body such as the back, chest, face and abdomen.

Basic Body Awareness in Therapy

An approach from Ogden enhances awareness of body and self through exploration of basic movement principles such as functional balance, free breathing, mental awareness and embodied presence (Ogden & Fisher, 2015). It involves both activating and experiencing the body through movement and acknowledging that these experiences touch different dimensions of existence:

- physical (like the organic matter of bones and muscles)
- physiological (processes such as blood circulation)
- psychological (attention, emotions)
- existential (the sense of "I am")

The body can be a starting point in the journey of healing. It is a repository of times of joy, loss and challenges. The multifaceted language of the body depicts all of those experiences. What we now know is that the body is able and willing to clearly communicate with us. What it takes, however, is a capacity and willingness to listen – and this refers to both therapist and client. That capacity and willingness can be nurtured and positively facilitated through experiential arts-based processes. Our body language is revealed in patterns of tension, movement, gesture, posture, breath, rhythm, facial expression, sensation, physiological arousal, gait and other action sequences (Ogden & Fisher, 2015, p. 14). A somatically oriented counsellor will take note of what they observe about a client's body-centred communication. Part of their work then is to support client exploration of bodily sensations to increase a client's awareness and feelings of safety in and with their own body.

One premise on which ET is grounded is that there is a natural intelligence of the body that can be tapped as a fundamental resource in clinical practice. Ogden's Sensorimotor Psychotherapy teaches clinicians to become interested in how the body carries the legacy of trauma and attachment inadequacies. Sensorimotor Psychotherapy aims to help clients change that legacy through somatic awareness and movement (Ogden & Fisher, 2015).

The ET Body Focus Activity

An ET Body Focus uses colours, shapes and words on a body outline as a resource for self-expression (see p. 139). The principle of the process is to map internal sensations and emotions on a body outline that is either pre-prepared or quickly sketched by the client. Under eight or nine years of age, the counsellor may prefer to quickly create the image on a large piece of art paper.

A creative arts activity, Body Focus enhances self-awareness, spatial awareness and supports reflection and articulation about somatic experiences and internal states. It can increase somatic sensitivity for a client, and may aid a counsellor in understanding, at a deeper level, a client's embodied experiences. Engaging in a body focus process offers a gentle, restorative tool for recovery from disconnection as well as helping a young client understand how they relate with their physical self, with others and with the world around them.

Body Focus activities invite a client to use colours, lines and shapes as a non-threatening approach to restore safe, tolerable connection with somatic experiences. A lived-body experience process, Body Focus means a client rehearses, in the safety of the therapeutic alliance, body and spatial awareness. This then supports a client to "listen" for information or meaning in body symptoms, in addition to helping them connect with bodily-held wisdom. Highly suitable for work with young clients, it teaches focus and body awareness through a simple activity to identify signals the body is under stress.

Body outline drawings that emerge from engagement in a Body Focus activity can provide a counsellor with useful data across time. The drawings will frequently chart a client's journey of re-connection with their body. The body outline drawings could also indicate emergence from dissociation of body experiences. In some cases, a client may find taking time to reflect on the images and narratives of their internal exploration enhances the inner-life skills of self-understanding and positive self-relating.

In addition to activities such as Body Focus, body scan, or a breathing activity, encouragement for a parent to offer hand, head or foot massage – where the counsellor assesses it is safe to do so – might help a young client feel they receive direct caregiver caring, time to re-connect with their body, and interpersonal support for a sense of relaxation.

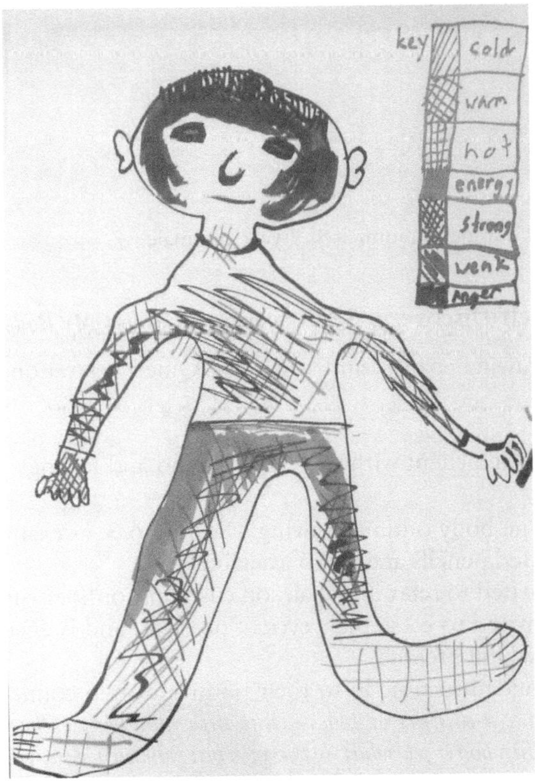

Figure 6.1 Body outline – 15-year-old male.

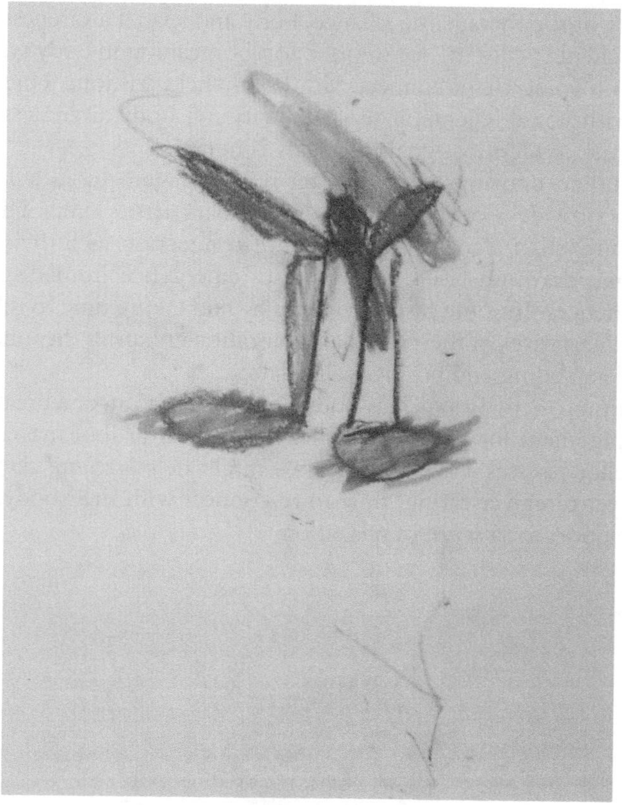

Figure 6.2 Body outline – traumatised 9-year-old male.

Activity 6.2 Self Discovery/Self-Awareness: *What My Body Tells Me*

Materials: Drawing paper and crayons. Quiet relaxation music in the background.

Aim: To re-orient a client with their body, mind and feelings.

1. Prepare large body outline drawing - See Fig 6.3. as example. Have crayons/coloured pencils and a pen available.
2. Client is invited to relax in a chair, on cushions, or floor rug if appropriate. Client is invited to close their eyes, if possible, and is encouraged to take several slow, full breaths.
3. Client is guided to tune in to their body and then connect to each part: *Can you take a minute or two to tune into your body? Check around on the inside of your body; see what is there; what you can discover. Begin in your head and move your attention gradually from your head down through your body to your toes.*

4. *See if you can pay attention as you search through your body and look for the different feelings I mention. If you find the feelings I am naming, record them on the body outline beside you. Pretend it is a map of you. See if you can use colours and lines to describe what you find.*

Then relax again, taking a breath and waiting for the next thing to look for.

If you do not find the feeling I name, breathe, relax and wait for the next search. Sometimes you might find the feeling in one part, sometimes several.

Take time to search for the thing mentioned. It could be found in your head, your shoulders, your arms and hands, your chest, belly, hips, legs and feet.

Take a big breath each time you relax and tune in and wait for the next search. (Use different ways to encourage the full breath.)

5. Search for six to eight of these: (counsellor chooses, but begins always with cool/cold followed by warm/hot as these are considered the most readily available states)
   - cool or cold
   - warm or hot
   - pain/pleasure
   - sadness/happiness
   - anger/loving
   - fear/courage
   - weakness/strength
   - disappointment/hope
   - tight, holding parts/relaxed, free, soft areas
   - agitated, upset or worried areas/peaceful parts
   - parts you don't like/favourite parts
   - place that feels like an animal, bird or fish might be. It could be resting, hiding or moving about.
6. Ask: *Is there anything else you've found inside that hasn't been mentioned?*
7. Beside the outline, take a couple of minutes to create a key code to show what was found.
8. After several searches, the body outline drawing is discussed. The client is invited to describe what was found and how they felt doing this exercise.
9. Encourage conversation that may:
   - enlarge on the client's self-awareness and
   - some possible causes for what was found (e.g.: feet hot after soccer practice).

Take some time to draw out connections between what was found in the body, what is happening in the client's life, and any emotions that may be linked.

10. Consider follow-up work indicated by what was found and indicated (see p. 140).

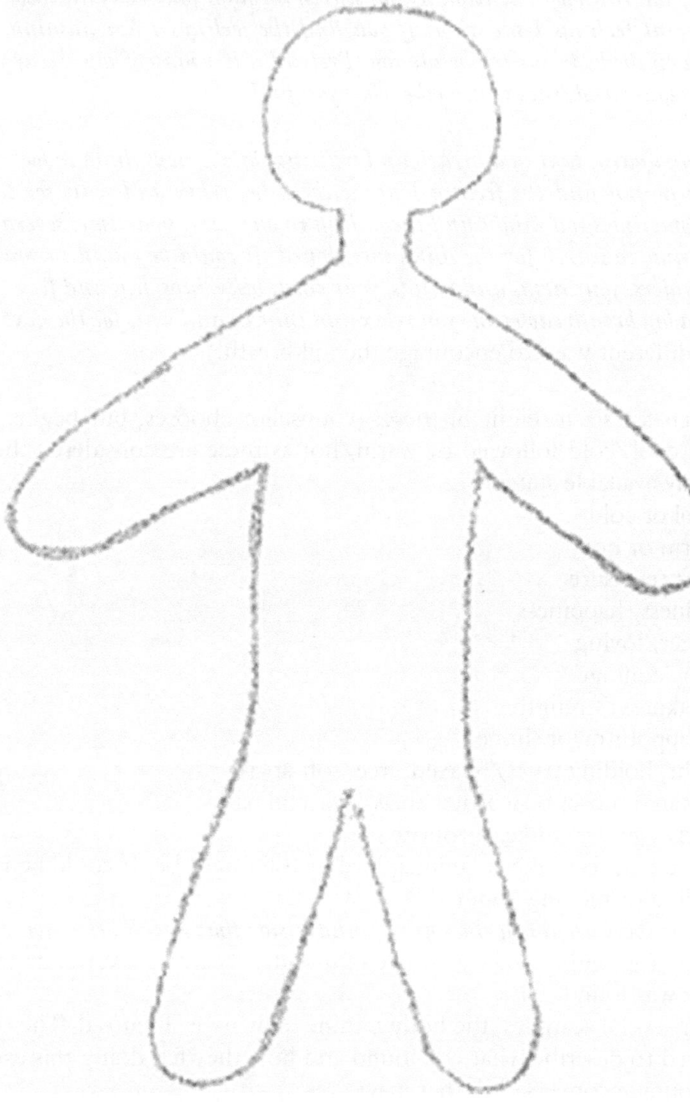

Figure 6.3 Worksheet – bad times / good times.

Aims and Follow-Up Strategies for Somatic Self-Awareness

The focus of ET activities that aim to enhance body awareness through:

- Awareness of tension
- Ability to notice any change in breathing when anxious or angry (shallow, deeper)
- Noticing emotional response to caring touch

- Can I feel the breath/sensation of breath travel in and out of the body?
- Can identify where in the body there is a physical response to emotion
- Can identify what might cause physical discomfort
- Able to take cues from the body.

Principles for Processing Body Symptoms

- Some somatic symptoms may be a sign that physical/emotional processing is needed and/or underway.
- There are two types of strategies that can be offered:
  - those that attempt to reduce or manage symptoms
  - those that process and can resolve the causes behind symptoms.

Both approaches can be appropriate at times, depending on your assessment of the level of emotional stability or wellbeing in the client.

- To begin exploring the causes of symptoms, involve:
  - the body
  - activate cognitive understanding/emotional intelligence
  - support connection with, and appropriate expression of, emotions.
- Safe, sustained awareness during an expressive intervention can allow some spontaneous resolution – similar to relaxation or meditation. The capacity of a young client for emotional processing is influenced not by chronology, but by emotional "age". Assessment of a client's emotional "age" prior to offering an ET activity is an important step.
- The meaning a client makes of any activity is what is of prime importance. There is benefit in regularly processing trauma symbolically and experientially so both the event and the experience can become emotionally tolerable and manageable. In using ET with a young client who has been traumatised, there is no requirement to rely on words or descriptions of actual events or feelings. Distress can be more obliquely communicated independent of words through choice of object, colour on the page, or even a piece of music.
- For the client who lives with the legacy of traumatic experience/s:

  a focus on talking about the trauma is often avoided; doing so activates a client's physiological state. The client's language is, or becomes, restricted and they may act in a "primitive way" as a form of protection for both themselves, and in cases where parental abuse is involved, protection for the parent through staying silent. The result can be an increase in anxiety. This means that verbal "therapy" alone may be ineffective – in the bigger picture. Integrating expressive work as a way to reorganise non-verbal and verbal recollections draws on a client's ability to function, activates their resilience and internal resources in ways that honour a young person's capacity to heal and grow.

Options for Body Focus Follow-Up Activities

- Post-exploration discussion and speculation on any information about causes of bodily experienced symptoms – as a way to encourage cognitive review and insight.
- Relaxation to reduce the effect of symptoms and use of sustained awareness.
- Bioenergetics, energy release activities, movement, or dance – to promote physical release.
- Body Focus activities – combining focused attention and relaxation with exploratory questions.
- Emotion-focused processes – these focus on contacting, processing and resolving underlying emotions.
- Role-play of images and symbols that accompany body symptoms – can bring resolution, insight and a reclaiming of positive qualities.

As the Support Person How Can I Help?

Understand the foundations of providing relational safety for a client, extend and deepen our capacity for providing a non-judgemental presence and increase our capacity and willingness to understand the language of the body.

Areas of awareness for therapist development:

- visual – *What do I observe in the client's bodily movement and expression?*
- auditory – *What is being said and how is it being said?*
- emotional – *What do I notice on an emotional level?*
- energetic – *What is the energetic quality of the experience?*
- somatic – *What do I feel in my own body?*

Activity 6.3 Integration through Role-play: *Messages from the Animal, Bird or Fish*

Aim: Use of metaphor to facilitate self-discovery; a safe, non-intrusive extension of bodily-held feelings exploration

Note: The counsellor guides the person into a role-play of the animal, bird or fish, and asks the following questions slowly, giving the client time to reflect and "feel" the answer, followed by giving a response to the counsellor's question. This activity can also be offered as a written activity if that is more appropriate for a client.

- Say to the client:
  - *Relax as much as you can and take a few deep breaths.*
  - *For this exercise can you pretend you are this animal, bird or fish?*
  - *Then with your permission, I would like to ask that animal, bird or fish some questions.*

- *If you are comfortable to do so, close your eyes, allow an image of what you found to come into your mind's eye.*
- *Be interested in all the aspects of the image, how it looks, feels and what its energy might be like.*
- *Now see if you can let yourself become this "symbol".*
- *Imagine your body changing; change your posture if it helps.*
- *Imagine the energy of this animal, bird or fish.*
- *Take some full breaths and feel how it would be to actually be it.*
- The client first imagines self as the symbol then answers these questions, responding with *"I"* rather than *"It"*.

1. *Can you tell me what you are?*
2. *Would you be able to describe what you look like?*
3. *Feel inside, can you tell me what you are made of, or what is inside you?*
4. *Could you describe any main feelings you are aware of?*
5. *What do you know about your age? Are you old or young? Can you tell me your age?*
6. *Do you have a sound or movement?*
   (If they do, ask them if they're able to describe/demonstrate the sound/movement)
7. *Do you have a special purpose?* (pause) *What are you for?*
8. *Is there anything you want?*
9. *Do you have a message for* ....(client's name), *or anything you would like to say to him/her? Any advice perhaps? Or any other comment?*

After a pause, say:

- *Now, taking one or two slow breaths, come back to being yourself, and then gently open your eyes.*
- *Did you hear that message?* (pause) *How does that feel?*

- After some discussion, encourage the client to write down the message so they have a record of it.
- Invite them to share how they feel after the exercise and to talk about any ways the message relates to or supports their life.
- Invite them to draw the animal, bird or fish and possibly add some words about its meaning for them.

Activity 6.4 Somatic Awareness: *My Belly Circle*

Materials: Crayons, A3 size drawing paper, large cushions to lean against.

Preparation: Client prepares a large circle on drawing paper.

Precautions: The appropriateness of this activity needs to be considered in the light of information about any physical or sexual abuse a client may have experienced.

Instructions

- *This activity is called "My Belly Circle". It may sound a little strange, but I am going to invite you to tune in and look inside, and see what you can find in the middle of your body, in your belly.*
- *Lean back on the cushions and relax as much as you can. Take some deep breaths.*

See if you can let your body go floppy for a moment.

Could you tune in to your belly now?

- *Feel what it's like from the inside.* (pause)
- *Is there a colour that goes with how it feels in the belly area?*
- *Is the colour the same all the way through?*
- *Or are there different areas? Is there one colour? Or more?*
- *Are there any areas where the colours are darker or lighter?*

- Client represents sensations by shading in colours in the circle, imagining the circle is their belly.
- *When you are ready, lean back again and relax.*

This time put your hands on your belly to help you tune in.
Take another deep, slow, full breath, as if you could breathe down deep.
Feel inside, tune in to your belly again:

- *Are there any shapes or lines that go with what's inside?*
- *Is it the same in the upper part as the lower part?*
- *Is it the same at each side – or different?* (pause)
- *Could you add any shapes or lines to the drawing that show how it feels in your belly at the moment?*

- Client draws shapes or lines representing the sensations, on top of the first colour(s).
- *As you look at your drawing:*
  - *Can you find a word or two that goes with what you experienced and drew in the circle?*
  - *Write the words on, or around, the drawing.*
  - *You can write them large or write them small.*
  - *See if you could add any words that go with how it feels inside.*
- Client leans back again, relaxes, takes a few deep, slow breaths, tunes into belly.
- *Imagine that sometimes your belly speaks in picture language as a way to talk to you:*
  - *From deep inside, your belly might send you a picture to show how it feels.*

    - *Watch in your mind for a picture that your belly might be sending at the moment.*
    - *There may be a picture; there may not.*
    - *If you can see a picture, sketch it at the edge of the drawing or on another page.*
- Client leans back again, tunes in to belly.
- *Imagine you have a microphone now.*
    - *You rest the microphone on your belly.*
    - *There is a cord from the microphone into a speaker that can turn belly language into people's language.*
    - *This speaker translates the sound inside into human words.*
    - *You have earphones too and perhaps can hear your belly speaking to you.*
    - *What is it saying? Is there something it wants to say to you?* (pause)

This could be just a few words or a sentence, or it could be silent.

Could you write down anything you might hear your belly telling you?

If you hear any words, could you write them beside or under the drawing, or on another page?

When you are ready, you can share your drawing with me, or keep it private; it is up to you.

Integration Discussion

- *Would you be willing to share with me what you've created on the page?*
- *How did it feel to do the activity?*
- *What did you discover in your belly? Were there any feelings or sensations in there?*
- *Is there anything your belly knows about your life?*
- *Could you sum up what you have discovered from this activity?*

Note: The same format can be used for the development of somatic awareness in other areas, e.g., legs and feet, hands, head, face, shoulders or chest.

Activity 6.5 Body Focus: *Expanding and Freeing Positive Energy*

Materials: Have crayons and paper ready.

Preparation: Ask client to prepare two large body outline drawings, with the titles: *Before* and *After*.

- Invite the client to relax as much as possible, lean back or lie down on some cushions. Again, suggest they relax and take a few slow, full breaths.

Instructions

- *Begin by feeling where your body rests on the cushion/carpet/in the chair. Let your body be heavy; feel what part of your back touches the carpet/chair. Slowly begin to move your awareness from your head down to your toes.*
- *You are invited to search inside your body to find any alive or excited parts. You are looking for alive energy, parts that feel warm, or parts of the body that you are more aware of.*
- *You may find one "alive" area or a few. Start to focus on one area that seems to feel most alive, excited or warm.*
- *Tune into it for a moment, then see what colour you would choose, what lines or shapes or shading would you create to go with the alive part.* (pause) *Allow yourself to create an image of it on the BEFORE body outline.*
- *Can you describe what you found? Are there any words you want to add to the image?*
- *Relax again and tune into the part that feels most alive. We are going to give this alive, excited energy a chance to reveal more about itself, its gifts.*
- *The questions I'm going to ask are for the excited, alive part. We are going to give it a chance to speak, to reveal itself, so you can learn more about yourself. Let the energy, the aliveness answer. You, the person, can relax and lend it your voice. Let it speak out the answers if it can.*

Wait for the answers to come. If there are no answers, that is OK.

So, here is the first question for that alive or excited energy:

- *Are you moving or still? flowing or held?*
- *How big are you? How far do you spread?*
- *Do you have a texture? Are you smooth or rough? Soft or bumpy? What do you feel like?*
- *How did you start? Do you remember when you began?*
- *Have you been there a long or a short time?*
- *Does the person you are in listen to you? Do they notice you?*
- *Is there anything you would like to say to the person you are with now?*
- *Is there a way that the body part that contains you would want to move?*
- *Could you let it happen now?*
  (Pause)
- *Is there any sound that wants to go with that?*
- *Is there a picture, image or symbol that goes with you?*
- *Send that picture to the mind of the person you are in.*
- *Imagine yourself expanding now, open out a little, let any movement help.*
- *Let the body support this image of expansion. See how that feels.* (pause)
- *What is the gift or the treasure you contain for this person?*
- *Do you have a name?*
- *Could you tell the person you are in the benefits and challenges of letting you free.*

- *silently or speak it out.*
- *Is there anything else you need to express now? Any advice for the person?*
- *Anything you want to make known?*

Take a slow full breath. Allow your attention to return to the room.

Completion and Integration

- The client draws how that part feels now onto the "after" body outline.
- Invite the client to compare the body outlines – invite them to notice and describe any differences.
- Invite them to create any image that the alive part presents.
- It might be helpful for them to write down what they have discovered from looking at the two body outlines.
- Is there any way this experience might relate to their current life?
- Invite the client to visualise and discuss creative ways of using times of aliveness.

Movement in Therapy

Movement can refer to the energy of motion inherent in emotions. Movement also acts as a catalyst for supporting mental processes in therapy. The first and foremost reason to incorporate movement in a counselling session with a young client is that movement is natural for them – sitting still for an hour is not. There is growing evidence that being sedentary can impact cognitive function and memory retention (e.g., Chandrasekaran et al., 2021; Chueh et al., 2022; Pindus et al., 2025)

The main types of movement used in ET include: Running around, imaginative role-play of animals, birds or fish, extremely slow movement to develop body awareness, structured movements such as bioenergetics and no movement – stillness. The therapist and client can experiment with movement as an expression of the client's inner world. Movement can offer a non-verbal means of communication. For instance, a counsellor might invite a client to make a gesture or take a stance that reflects or represents how they are feeling in the moment. The counsellor might then ask the client to exaggerate that gesture, in order to heighten the experience, to connect more fully with the body and the joy of movement.

It can be useful to take some time to observe how our clients use their bodies. Watch for any characteristic body stance. Body postures can reflect ongoing emotional states. Emotional stances, physical postures, may be habitual or the result of a temporary state. Making these stances conscious in our clients can provide more choice in addressing the somatic component of mood.

Common denominators of typical body postures seem to be contraction or expansion, closeness or openness. Positive feelings and stances tend to go with an expanded body; negative feelings are usually reflected in some contraction in the physical presentation.

Activity 6.6 Somatic Experiencing: *Exploring Body Postures*

Aim: Provides experience of several common body postures that have associated emotional states and self-beliefs. It develops the skill of "watching" these postures from the inside.

Instructions

Guide the client to take the postures that go with the emotional states listed below, one at a time. They are invited to close their eyes if they are comfortable to do so, and hold each posture, then allow awareness of their internal experience.

Say to the Client

- Take a moment to turn your focus towards your body – "looking in". Take a steady, deep breath and bring your awareness to inside yourself at this moment.
- I'm going to invite you to take some postures and suggest you try this with your eyes closed at first.
- The aim is to explore how each posture feels from the inside. See which muscles are used.
- Feel right through your body – how you experience the posture in each part of your body, as if you were taking an internal photograph.
- After a moment, I will suggest you open your eyes and see what the posture looks like from the outside.
- Watch to see if any of these are familiar to you. Particularly notice what happens in the transitions between body postures.
- Now see if you can find a body posture that goes with these statements, and repeat the statements as you take the posture:
  - I'm sad. I'm very sad.
  - I'm feeling good. I'm so happy right now!
  - Leave me alone. I'm better alone, by myself.
  - I feel open. I'm happy to be close to others now.
  - I'm really a loser. It's happening again. Nothing goes right for me.
  - Everything gets better and better all the time. I feel like a winner!
  - They do it to me. It's their fault. I'm a victim.
  - I am a hero/heroine! No challenge is too great. I'm safe and strong.
- Was there one of these body postures that feels more familiar? One you know well, one with the most emotional "charge" to it? Could you make that particular posture again?
- Take a full breath. Take the posture again. Feel what your body is doing. Exaggerate the posture.
- Now allow yourself to move a little with it. See if there is any sound or words that go with it.
- Take a moment to check inside your body. See what you can connect with.
- Is there any sense of energy flowing or moving at the moment?

- Could there be any emotional message for you from that posture? What might your body be saying to you right now?
- Would you be willing to share something of your experience of exploring body postures?

Activity 6.7 Movement for Somatic Awareness: *Slow-Motion Snails*

Aim: To work with focused attention, to connect with the body and let it loosen, relax and connect with the energy inside.

Resources: To begin, have quiet, relaxing music in the background. Have rhythmic music available for Step 9.

Instructions: Begin with simple centring through inviting a client to take two or three steady breaths with their attention on the breath moving in and out of their body. The client is then invited to stand in a way so their body feels relaxed, or less tense.

1. **Neck**: Eyes closed, or gaze softened. Let your neck relax, allow your chin to move slowly down towards your chest. Do it very slowly, feel each degree of "let-go". Imagine you can be in the muscles. Include continual letting-go in the whole body and sighing the breath out fully.
2. **Arms**: Slowly raise your arms up in front of you until they are about level with your shoulders, then slowly let go. Wrists are loose. Feel the use of tension as they rise and the degrees of letting go as they flow down again.
3. **Knees**: Slowly bend your knees. Keep some awareness in the centre of you. Feel the "let-go" as the body goes down and the adding on of strength as you rise up. Keep the rest of the body more or less straight but not rigid!
4. **Arms and Knees**: Let arms and knees move together now. The arms rising as the knees bend down. Each time you come up, feel the tall point. Keep allowing breath to release. Keep it slow.
5. **Wrists and Palms**: Allow free-flowing movement in arms – they move by themselves. Then add tension slowly through the hand as arms go down, bending hands back at the wrists. As arms rise, wrists are loose; as arms let go, wrists are tensed. This tension is felt through the palms of the hands.
6. **Arms, Wrists and Knees**: Let arms, wrists and knees flow together. There is no "right" way; you cannot make a mistake. If you get confused, simply begin again with just the arms, then add knees and wrists one at a time.
7. **Arms, Wrists, Knees, Neck**: Continue, then add the neck if possible. The neck goes down as arms rise. Keep it slow!
8. Try Steps 1–7 separately, then, to the other movements, add a turning of the torso to the side as arms rise and a return to the centre as arms flow down. First to the right, then to the left. If it all goes astray – the client can relax and start again.

9. Let the head free and flow into free dance or movement. Invite interest in how the body wants to respond to the music.
10. Finding stillness – The client is invited to rest, lie down, or sit quietly in a chair. Invite them to feel what it is like on the inside now.

Playing with Breath

Without our conscious intent, the respiratory system can become involved in protection from difficult feelings, primarily by diminishing the depth or fullness of breaths. Shallower breathing, with muscular tension across the chest, appears to help create distance from experiencing emotion. Taking deeper and fuller breaths, allowing the lungs to expand, is in a way like saying "Yes" to being in contact with emotions and letting them flow. Breath has been used in counselling and psychotherapy over the ages to assist with healing (Caldwell & Victoria, 2011). Varying breathing speed and depth is used in yoga to either stimulate energy or bring a calming effect. Breathing games are a gentle and fun way to support young clients to make deeper contact with themselves and release some emotional and physiological constriction.

One caution with breathing games relates to the early 2000s global experience of the COVID-19 pandemic. Safety of participants' health is paramount – whether they participate in a group or an individual session. Before offering breathing exercises, please consider the wellbeing of yourself and your client/s, the space available (indoors or outdoors), as well as any health cautions or warnings from any regulatory agencies.

Between, during and after each part of each activity, it can be helpful to encourage some deep breaths. This will help clients connect with themselves and begin to feel more "open". As the therapist, we take time to notice a client's breathing. Some appear to be holding their breath – perhaps a learned response to fear or apprehension – perhaps waiting for a signal that life is safe, so they can start to breathe (feel) again.

Activity 6.8 Breathing Games

Aims: These games are designed to activate energy and stimulate emotion through strong breathing. They can be used as preparation for emotional release processes and as a way to help young clients de-stress. Spend some time setting the scene before each exercise. Consider carefully the cultural appropriateness of each game, and creatively adapt if, and as, appropriate.

The Rabbit

- Client imagines self as a rabbit jumping around a sunny field enjoying a lunch of long, lush green grass.
- Suddenly a fox appears, the rabbit freezes, holding its breath.

- Then it dashes home to their safe burrow and sits, panting quickly for a while.
- (Repeat)

The Horse

- Client imagines themselves as a horse. If space is available, they can be invited to "gallop" around the room.
- They are told it is a very cold morning, and this horse is snorting very strongly, so strongly that you can see the breath.
- They become the snorting horse, galloping over the hills.
- How far does the breath extend as they breathe out? Imagine seeing the breath.

More Breathing Game Suggestions

- Be a whale coming to the surface of the ocean and exhaling powerfully – imagine a fine spray of water bursting out. Then, breathe in, hold, imagine diving down deep, then surfacing again.
- Become a dragon breathing fire – how far can you send the flames?
- Blow up some large imaginary balloons.
- Blow bubbles – keep bubbles going as long as possible.

Giving Instructions to Breathe More Fully

- Vary the ways of giving the instruction to take deep breaths so that it does not become boring or mechanical.
- Emphasise relaxation on the out-breath.
- When sitting or lying down:
  - *Place your hand on your chest. Does your chest feel tight/held, or willing to expand?*
  - *Take a big breath and let it out. How does that feel? How much does your chest move?*
  - *Can you breathe in so much air that your lungs feel huge?*
  - *Place your hands on your rib cage, feel what happens as you empty out all your breath.*
  - *Take a breath in through your nose. Let the air out through your mouth.*
  - *Take three fast breaths – in and out.*
  - *Take a big breath in through your right nostril and let the air out through your left. Then in through the left, and out the right.* (Using your finger may help.)
  - *Take a big breath very, very slowly. How slowly could you breathe in?*
  - *Take six slow, big breaths as if you were a balloon being blown up:*
    - *Take in a breath with each number I count. 1, 2, 3,* etc.
    - *After 6, let the breath out with some noise, as if someone suddenly let the balloon go!*

Activity 6.9 Exploring Somatic Communication: *Speaking without Words*

Aims: This activity can support grounding and can be useful for clients who may not be ready to express themselves verbally.

Instructions

Explore, try out, some gestures that go with these statements:

- *Keep away*
- *Come close*
- *Getting ready for school*
- *Saturday mornings*

Could you share a little about how each posture felt to you?

The ET Adaptation of Bioenergetics

> *A fundamental thesis of bioenergetics is that the body and mind are functionally identical: That is, what goes on in the mind reflects what is happening in the body and vice versa.*
>
> Lowen and Lowen (2003)

Dr Alexander Lowen (1910–2008) was a student of Wilhelm Reich. Reich is considered one of the grandfathers of body-oriented therapies. Lowen was the Founder/creator of bioenergetics, with its focus on awareness, breathing, centring, grounding, feeling, movement. Bioenergetics consists of a collection of physical activities that include breathing, grounding, breathing with movement, stretching, shaking as well as expressive movements, that may be accompanied by evocative vocal expressions.

Bioenergetic therapy was based on exercises developed in the USA in the 1960s by two psychiatrists, Alexander Lowen and John Pierrakos, both of whom had been students and colleagues of Wilhelm Reich.

Wilhelm Reich (1889–1957), an Austrian doctor and psychoanalyst, was a member of the second generation of psychoanalysts after Freud. His idea of muscular armouring – the expression of the personality in the way the body moves – shaped innovations such as body psychotherapy, gestalt therapy, bioenergetic analysis and primal therapy. Reich's contributions to understanding how the breathing and muscular systems are connected in habitual patterns are valuable and have been incorporated into many different modern therapies (Gilbert, 1999).

His message of sexual liberation was experienced as disturbing by the psychoanalytic community. His vegetotherapy, in which he massaged his disrobed patients to dissolve their "muscular armour", violated the key taboos of psychoanalysis and therapy in general. Reich coined the term "orgone" for a biological energy he said he had discovered, which he claimed others called God. Reich was unaware of the many thousands of years of study of the human energy system in Chinese medicine, yet his work illuminated similar concepts.

Recommended Literature

Lowen, A., & Lowen, L. (2003). *The way to vibrant health – A manual of bioenergetics.* Bioenergetics Press.
Lowen, A. (1994). *Bioenergetics: The revolutionary therapy that uses the language of the body to heal the problems of the mind.* Bioenergetic Press.

Ideally, the body, mind and feelings work in flow together. What is denied or excluded from awareness, or what we refrain from expressing, gets "stuck". This lack of flow is expressed through ongoing muscular tension or what Reich called "armouring". Chronic muscular tension is connected with negative and destructive thoughts and attitudes, which can translate into negative and destructive actions. For emotional and physical wellbeing, feelings and energy need to return to a flowing state of freedom, beauty and grace.

Bioenergetics mobilises physical energy as well as emotional energy. Bioenergetics can be used to "let off steam" as well as prepare for a more gentle and deeper connection with emotions. The outcome can depend on the duration and intent of the activities. Many of the bioenergetic activities and games use intentional tension to mobilise and stretch the muscles to help body armouring relax. Bioenergetics are helpful for clients who report feeling depressed or who have contained their feelings, or restricted access to their emotional life, although they may initially feel worse. An atmosphere of fun and use of rhythm and imagery will help wholehearted participation.

Clients are reminded not to take part in any posture that is painful for the body – there is no "endurance" involved in bioenergetics in the ET style. Adolescents may resist anything that seems to make them appear silly. Counsellors should explore the bioenergetic activities personally and participate energetically in them, model them enthusiastically – and be prepared to look a bit silly!

Activity 6.10 Bioenergetic Activities: *Using Tension to Enhance Self-Awareness*

Materials: Prepare drawing materials and a circle for mandala completion drawing. Have gentle relaxing music available for later quiet stages.

Aim: To heighten body awareness and body self-compassion.

Note: Provide a brief spoken introduction to some basic principles of bioenergetics.

Standing

- **Tension in Arms**: Explore the effect of tension in arms and hands – one arm and hand are stretched forward, then relaxed; compare awareness of arms *"What do you notice there?"*, then work with the other arm.
- **Bound and Free**: Cross legs, wrap arms around body, tighten body gradually from toes up to head, hold tension and breath, burst free and shake body, running on the spot. Repeat three times.
- **Face**: Tighten eyes and jaw, hold, take a big breath in and hold it, release breath and open eyes and jaw wide, blink and move jaw a little.
- **Shoulders**: Very slowly bring shoulders up towards the ears, hold tension, hold breath, drop shoulders, release breath, shiver and shake shoulders.
- **Arms**: Bring hands together, fingers touching, turn fingers in facing towards the chest, extend arms out away from the chest to create tension, push wrists away from the chest, hold tension, breathe, then soften, relax and repeat.
- **The Star**: Feet apart, relax knees, stretch out arms and fingers, allow upper body to open, lean back, open chest, stretch arms and fingers out wide, as far back as possible, hold briefly, let go, repeat three times.
- **The Arch, or Bow** (as in bow and arrow): A basic stress position, bend knees, rest hands gently on lower back, open chest, leaning back slowly, without letting head drop back, until the whole front of the body feels open. Breathe deeply and slowly, allow any stress or vibrations in muscles to build up. Alternate with bending forward and shaking gently, going floppy.

Lie Down and Relax

- **Heart Opening**: Relax in a chair or on some floor cushions with your back over a large cushion, so that the chest is in an open position. Bring awareness to the breath, relax and allow a sense of opening.
- (Use gentle background music)
- **Energy in Legs**: From lying position, stretch each leg, imagine it is growing longer, let the leg respond to the image, then relax. Alternate legs, then rest. Keep focus on energy in legs.
- **Rest with Inner Focus**: From lying position, tune in to the energy in the whole body, be still. Remain aware of how the body feels and how the energy within and around it feels.

Sit and Draw

- **Mandala**: In a circular framework, draw lines, colours, shapes or images that go with how you feel now. Is there a word or two that goes with how you feel inside now?
- **Discussion**: The client is invited to share how they found the activities and how they feel now.

Activity 6.11 Bioenergetic Activities: *Releasing Frustration and Reclaiming Strength*

Materials: Large cushions for hitting and kicking at, drawing materials. Background music – with clear rhythm to support or encourage movement. Strong energetic music for Step 4 may help.

Aim: Using metaphor and imagery to support the release of blocked physical energy and expression of emotion in a way that helps the activity seem playful and light-hearted. Support the flow of positive energy.

1. Shaking

Ask the client to *"Imagine you are a dog or a polar bear. You have been swimming. You come out of the water. Do you remember how to shake off the water? Loosen your body, shake, in turn, your head, shoulders, arms, back, hips, legs. Take some deep breaths. Try shaking all of yourself"*.

2. Discuss Any Resistance

How did you feel about that? E.g., Was it a bit embarrassing? fun? weird?

3. "Get Off My Back!"

Make fists, bring arms up in front of your body so your elbows are level with your shoulders. Open out, moving your elbows back as far as possible. Move elbows together, then separately. Add the words: Get off my back!

4. Anger Role-Play

Pretend you are an actor auditioning for a part you are keen to get in a film or play. Maybe you think this could lead to an Academy Award! It is the role of someone who is very angry. Find a way to stand that goes with "I am furious!" Add hand movements. Find a facial expression that goes with the angry feeling, then exaggerate it all. When the music comes on, let the actor play the part – moving and speaking and making sounds.

5. Wood-Chopper

Your feet are apart, your knees are bent a little. Your hands are clasped together and stretched back over your head. This creates tension, and then you swing your hands down in front of you, releasing the tension in your back. Allow your strength to come from low in your body, through your back. Add some power sounds! Do not do this if you have a back/arm or leg injury.

6. Boxer in Training

Have you seen one of the "Rocky" movies? Imagine you are a boxer in training. Start your air-punching practice, start slowly, build up speed and strength, add some deep breaths, explore power sounds, alternate arms. (A large cushion can also be used to hit into.)

7. Kicking

release through the legs into a strong pillow. *Aim for the middle, find your power sound. Keep going till you want to stop. Start slow, build up speed and strength.*

8. Walking

Walk around the room, relax hips, let-go in shoulders, let it flow.

9. Step Forward

While walking: *Step forward with strong, firm steps that show: "I am here! This is me!"*

Integration:

Stand Still

Tune into your body now. Feel what is happening inside. (pause) *Allow an image from nature to come into your mind, a picture of something from nature that goes with your energy now.* (pause) *Picture it in your mind. Feel its three main qualities or strengths. For a moment, pretend you are that thing from nature.*

- Brief *role-play* with the symbol.

  Say *"I am a …"*
  "My main strengths are …"

- Invite the client to:
  - *draw* the symbol from nature
  - add *words* for its three main qualities or strengths that emerged
  - *write down* what they learnt from the activity
- **Discuss**: *Is there a time or place in your life when these qualities or strengths would be useful?*

Activity 6.12 Bioenergetics: *Letting Go of Sadness and Grief*

Materials: Drawing materials ready.

Aim: The work with bioenergetic release is based on the need to reconnect the flow of energy between body, mind and feelings. Bioenergetic activities focus on the importance of the young person feeling grounded. The focus is that blocks to emotional expression and wellbeing can be expressed through the body.

Music: Quiet relaxing music for the last four steps (e.g., *Mariner, Secret Garden*).

Warm Up: Shaking, holding the whole body tight, breaking free with running, shaking and sound.

The Arch: Feet apart, knees bent, hands resting gently on lower back, lean back to open chest, do not let the head fall back, until eyes are facing the ceiling. Hold the stressed position for a while, then relax, slowly come upright, lean forward and allow your spine to open. Alternate arch and forward flop about three or four times.

Freeing Up the Face:

- rolling eyes – head still, make large circles with eyeballs
- eyes tight shut, breath held – burst open, breath out with sound – repeat four times
- alternate: happy face/sad face – exaggerate these – repeat
- imitate crying, then laughing – repeat
- In front of a mirror: make horrible monster faces. Add some sounds that go with the faces.

Shoulder Rolls: Make large circles with shoulders, then shake and shiver
Get Off My Back: Focus on opening the front of the chest, arms up – elbows level with shoulders, fists tight, open out. Then one shoulder at a time with any words that want to be expressed.
Surrender: Growing taller on in-breath, then let-go, relax on each out-breath: relax neck, then on the next out-breath relax shoulders, then belly, finally knees, then repeat.
The Fern: Sit cross-legged on a cushion, swaying, releasing all breath with a sigh, focus on loosening hips. *Swaying like a fern in a gentle breeze that keeps changing directions.*
If there is space on the floor and it feels comfortable to do so, let yourself lie down on the floor.
Reaching Out: Arms are reaching up to the ceiling. Allow your breath to be free and open. Wait and see if any words or feelings come into your mind or heart.
Tuning-In: Lying down – deep surrender for a moment – *Feel your energy now.*
Fat and Thin: Lying down, diaphragm breathing, right hand on chest, left hand over belly, expand chest on in-breath, on out-breath let the belly expand. Imagine breath flowing down to your belly.

Melting: Lying down – breathe fully. Breathe in – hold breath in for a moment, then relax the whole body on out-breath, imagine the whole body melting onto the carpet on the out-breath.
Tune In: To feelings and energy in the chest. *What colours, lines, shapes or pictures would go with the energy in your chest?*

The client is invited to use the mandala shape to ***draw*** how they feel in the chest area.

Activity 6.13 Bioenergetic Games: *Releasing Stress*

Preparation: Have some rhythmic background music ready (e.g., *Exotic Dance* – Track 1)

Note: De-brief as you go if it helps the client feel more comfortable.

- Counsellor models each game first, then interacts with the client:
- **The Over-Packed Suitcase**:
  - Take turns to push each other down – hands on shoulders from behind, add pressure.
  - The one being pushed down is the suitcase, which suddenly springs up and breaks free, with a loud sound, and imagine all the clothes bursting out of the suitcase.
- **Tug of War**:
  - Pull on a rolled towel (or link hands) to activate strength, and use the whole body.
  - Do not let go!
  - At first, the client thinks either *NO* or *YES* while pulling,
  - Then after a while they whisper, then speak the words out loud.
  - Then let the *YES* or *NO* be all through the body.
- **Standing Hand-to-hand**: (or *How Strong Is the Wall?)*
  - Client and counsellor gradually mobilise their strength through pushing.
  - Gradually activate as many muscles of the body as possible,
  - from feet up to hands, push towards the other.
  - After a while, go floppy – at the same time.
- **Air Kicks**:
  - Alternating feet, kick into the air, let the kicks build up in strength.
  - Power sounds, words, or phrases can be added after a while.
  - Client is encouraged to keep kicking until they tire.
- **The Victory "YES!"**:
  - This is like a punch, but with a downward motion, closing fist "taking hold of strength".
  - Take a firm step forward each time, alternating hands and feet.
  - Accompany each step with exclaiming a loud "Yes!"
  - Briefly ponder: *What are the strengths you are saying YES to?*
- **Walk Vigorously**:

- Move around the room for a minute – taking long steps.
- Relax, and let shoulders and hips move freely.

- **Rest**:
  - *Tune in to your body, your energy, mood. What are you aware of? How do your legs feel now? Your arms? Tummy? Chest?*
  - Client is invited to draw how they feel with either a mandala or a body outline, or write down what they have noticed.
  - Invite the client to discuss how they felt during and after the games.

Moving Towards Relaxation

Various types of relaxation are represented in the activities in this book, such as progressive relaxation (similar to Jacobson's sequential contraction and relaxation of major muscle groups [1929, cited in Lusebrink, 1990]), use of imagery – e.g., a rag doll, melting cheese on a pizza (similar to Schultz's Autogenic Training which uses images of warmth and heaviness to invoke relaxation [in Lusebrink, 1990]). The importance of the "let it happen" attitude to relaxation and the passive concentration on the breathing recommended by Schultz in Autogenic Training (Benson & Klipper, 2000) also reflects the approach to relaxation adopted here.

Relaxation can be used as a basis for developing sensory awareness and has proved useful in supporting clients' therapeutic process. Relaxation is introduced to clients to enhance their self-care skills base and is used in sessions as an integration process, particularly after expressive work with emotions.

Relaxation training has proved useful over time in many fields of endeavour (Carlson & Hoyle, 1993; Goldfried & Trier, 1974; Ost, 1987). Biophysical methods using muscle relaxation have added to the success of cognitive-behavioural approaches for many years (Rosenberg et al., 1997).

Relaxation therapy is evidence-based and was found to be efficacious, non-invasive and cost-efficient (Lovas, 2015). Lovas' review of the research highlighted that relaxation can maintain health and wellbeing amid the rapid change and chronic stress of today's society. Relaxation training improved sleep quality and cognitive function in people aged 60 years or older, and anxiety was reduced by relaxation techniques in hospitalised patients and people with cancer. Depression was reduced in caregivers, in women with breast cancer, people with chronic fatigue, post-traumatic stress disorder and adolescent psychiatric patients. Relaxation reduced nightmares, depression, sleep disturbances and dissociation in trauma-exposed individuals and improved post-surgical wound healing. Relaxation is a practical skill that needs to be performed regularly to be effective (Lovas, 2015).

Benson and Klipper (2000) refer to the extensive medical research on the value of relaxation and describe the inherent relaxation response as an "innate mechanism within us". The key ingredients that support this relaxation response are a quiet environment, the use of a mental device, a passive attitude and a physically comfortable position.

Holian (2001) found the use of ET creative visualisations highly effective as an adjunct in supporting student relaxation, as well as increasing concentration. A school-based relaxation training programme reduced students' stress and anxiety levels, and can be used as a preventative strategy (Morton & Cescato, 2000).

Autogenic Relaxation Training (self-directed use of relaxation imagery) has proved to be effective in reducing anxiety and depression in some health conditions (Vasu et al., 2020). It was beneficial in reducing anxiety and depression, and improving functional ability, mobility and quality of life among stroke survivors.

Music assisted relaxation can lower systolic blood pressure of patients with diabetes and a comorbidity of hypertension (Mandel et al., 2013). Relaxation therapy is effective in reducing PTSD severity, anxiety and depression symptoms, and to improve quality of life (Carletto et al., 2016). The level of students' anxiety when facing a test was decreased after participating in group counselling activities with relaxation techniques, assisted by music (Nurlela & Jannati, 2019). Results revealed a significant reduction in stress for university students, with medium to large effect sizes during their first visit to participate in a self-guided relaxation zone programme (Jones et al., 2023). An optimal dose of self-guided relaxation ranged from two to eight visits to the relaxation zone.

Creating a Relaxation Sequence

You can follow these typical stages when constructing or modifying your own relaxation sequences:

Before:

- Set the workspace – make it private, dimmed lights help eyes relax, create order.
- maybe have an attractive focus area. Prepare expression/integration materials: paper, crayons, clay, writing materials, etc.
- Present an overview of the sequence – and give a brief rationale. Normalise mind-wandering and find metaphors for this.
- Address any trust or safety issues: Is there any apprehension, resistance or self-consciousness?

During:

- Use invitational language and offer options. Pose questions rather than statements. Avoid saying *"Now I want you to …"* Say: *"See if you could …"* or *"See if you would like to …"*

1. Release of agitation, excitement, nervousness, e.g., brisk walking, shaking, bioenergetics, breathing games and sounding.

2. Somatic awareness as a starting point. Tuning-in to "what is there" at first – without a need to change anything. Guide attention to focus on body sensations, mood and energy level.
3. Structure the relaxation sequence to give a sense of order. For example: Is it for the whole body, or for parts? Is the sequence moving around the limbs? Or through the centre of the body?
4. Use language that can convey relaxation; imagery can help convey the sense of letting go, e.g.: *"floppy like a puppy asleep", "soft like melted cheese on a pizza". "like a gentle breeze". "Like fluffy clouds on a warm day"*, etc.
5. Support mindful focus; guide the client's attention and gently call it back when distracted.
6. Does the sequence use a visualisation, a story or a journey? Are there "signposts" along the way? Is there a safe, enjoyable place? Will you incorporate a "return" journey after Step 8?
7. It is useful to use imagery in the visualisation to support body awareness, e.g., use an array of senses.
8. Stillness and silence – Ensure there is some time in the sequence where nothing is said or done, where there is stillness and silence. The length of this time will depend on the client's attention span.
9. Gently, gradually, reconnecting with the room and outside world.
10. Private expression and recording of experiences: Suggest a range of options, e.g., drawing, writing, modelling, choosing miniatures to represent the experience, etc.

After:

- Sharing of experiences: Offer reflection questions.
- Assess from the discussion and artwork any need for follow-up; have any "doorways" to the client's process opened?

Activity 6.14 Expression Game: *Child/Parent Role-Play*

Client and counsellor face each other – choose roles: One is the parent, the other is the child.

- "Parent" says with a stern face: *"Be quiet!" "Come back here!"* etc., and cannot move from the spot.
- The "child" rebels: *"No! You can't make me!"* etc., and moves about, making lots of noise.
- Then swap words/roles.

Integration

If finishing the session after this game, integrate by resting, visualising colours, words or images from nature that go with how they feel now. Then draw how they feel inside, and then discuss the activity.

If continuing with a relaxation, leave integration and discussion till later in the session.

Activity 6.15 Relaxation Activity: *Tension and Surrender – The Star*

Aim: A relaxation and grounding activity to release tensions and support centring. It is supportive to use before quiet relaxation work. It uses over-stressing to assist a deeper relaxation. Ideal for young people who are not ready for quiet, still relaxation work.

Instructions

- Provide a brief explanation of, and reason for, the activity.
- The client lies on their back on a carpeted floor and stretches out their limbs.
- The client is asked to tune in to somatic sensations.
- Next the client is invited to contract and expand their whole body a few times, and then relax and be still.
- Client visualises self: As a five-pointed star, with each limb and the head as a point, floating, twinkling in a clear night sky.

They are asked to make their body into this star shape.

Say: *Now the star is going to try some exercises to help it twinkle!*
Begin tightening the muscles of your body, in this order:
right hand, right arm, hold for a moment, let go;
right foot, right leg, hold for a moment, let go;
left foot, left leg, hold for a moment, let go;
left hand, left arm, hold for a moment, let go;
face, trunk, hold for a moment, let go.
Work around the limbs about six to eight times.
Establish a rhythm: *Tense! Tense! Hold! Relax!*

(In group work you can use a drum beat to help establish the rhythm.)

Invite client to focus internally, and say:
See if you can be still now.
Can you feel inside? How does it feel inside you now?

(Pause)

- *What colours and lines and shapes would go with how it feels inside?*
- The client is invited to draw how they feel.
- Discussion is encouraged on:
- how they felt before, during and after the activity
- any creative projects they would enjoy participating in.

Activity 6.16 Relaxation, Grounding and Mindfulness: *Slow Walking*

Materials: paper and crayons.

Aim: Support for enhanced mindful somatic focus; generate relaxation, mindfulness and feelings of stillness.

Notes: Counsellor could participate with the client. Having bare feet may enhance the effectiveness.

Preparation: Client stands on the art paper and traces around their feet.

Warm-up: Quick walking, stomping, jumping, massaging feet.

1. Client walks slowly around the room, in a large circle. Counsellor brings these questions slowly, with pauses:
   - *Tune in to your feet. Begin to feel the floor under your feet.*
   - *Relax your whole body as much as you can.*
   - *Can you let your neck relax?*
   - *Allow your shoulders to drop. Let your arms swing free.*
   - *Let some full breaths flow in.*
   - *Allow your belly to be as soft as it can.*
   - *Tune in to your knees. Be aware of your knees. How are they? What do you notice?*
   - *Now slow down your walking. Keep walking, but slowly now.*
   - *Can you walk and relax your ankles at the same time?*
   - *Take three large slow breaths and let the breath relax out.*
   - *Become aware of your feet, feel how your toes, sole and heels touch the floor as you walk.*
   - *Which part of your feet touches the floor first?*
   - *Can you practise walking and feeling your feet from the inside for a while?*
2. The counsellor can decide whether the conditions would make it suitable to walk outside and walk in bare feet. If walking in bare feet, choose a path which provides different textures for the feet to experience.
   - Direct the client's attention to sensations in the feet, to differences in: Texture, temperature, hardness/softness underfoot.
   - Remind the client to bring their attention back inside themselves to feel their feet.
3. Clients are asked to stop, close their eyes and stand still for a moment and feel the earth under their feet. Are their feet warm or cool? Are there areas that are easier to be aware of? Areas that connect with the floor/earth?
4. Draw: Client uses colours and lines on the prepared feet outlines to express the sensations they felt in the feet.

5. Discuss

    - what has been expressed in the feet outlines
    - what it felt like to walk this way
    - anything they noticed while participating in the activity
    - how they feel after the activity.

References

Benson, H., & Klipper, M. Z. (2000). *The relaxation response*. Harper Collins.

Caldwell, C., & Victoria, H. K. (2011). Breathwork in body psychotherapy: Towards a more unified theory and practice. *Body, Movement and Dance in Psychotherapy*, *6*(2), 89–101.

Carletto, S., Borghi, M., Bertino, G., Oliva, F., Cavallo, M., Hofmann, A., & Ostacoli, L. (2016). Treating post-traumatic stress disorder in patients with multiple sclerosis: A randomized controlled trial comparing the efficacy of eye movement desensitization and reprocessing and relaxation therapy. *Frontiers in Psychology*, *7*, Article 526.

Carlson, C. R., & Hoyle, R. H. (1993). Efficacy of abbreviated progressive muscle relaxation training: A quantitative review of behavioural medicine research. *Journal of Consulting and Clinical Psychology*, *61*(6), 1059–1067.

Chandrasekaran, B., Pesola, A. J., Rao, C. R., & Arumugam, A. (2021). Does breaking up prolonged sitting improve cognitive functions in sedentary adults? A mapping review and hypothesis formulation on the potential physiological mechanisms. *BMC Musculoskeletal Disorders*, *22*(1), 1–16.

Chueh, T. Y., Chen, Y. C., & Hung, T. M. (2022). Acute effect of breaking up prolonged sitting on cognition: A systematic review. *BMJ Open*, *12*(3), e050458.

Damasio, A. (2003). Feelings of emotion and the self. *Annals of the New York Academy of Sciences*, *1001*(1), 253–261.

Gilbert, C. (1999). Breathing: The legacy of Wilhelm Reich. *Journal of Bodywork and Movement Therapies*, *3*(2), 97–106.

Goldfried, M. R., & Trier, C. S. (1974). Effectiveness of relaxation as an active coping skill. *Journal of Abnormal Psychology*, *83*(4), 348–355.

Gyllensten, A. L., Jacobsen, L. N., & Gard, G. (2019). Clinician perspectives of Basic Body Awareness Therapy (BBAT) in mental health physical therapy: An international qualitative study. *Journal of Bodywork and Movement Therapies*, *23*(4), 746–751.

Gyllensten, A. L., Skär, L., Miller, M., & Gard, G. (2010). Embodied identity: A deeper understanding of body awareness. *Physiotherapy Theory and Practice*, *26*(7), 439–446.

Holian, L. (2001). *Metacognition: Highlighting the importance of emotional reflection and expression* (Unpublished master's project). Monash University.

Jones, V. L., Salgado García, F. I., Brewer, L. M., Pérez-Muñoz, A., Schenck, L. A. M., You, Z., & Andrasik, F. (2023). The relaxation zone: Initial analysis of stress management services for university students. *Journal of American College Health*, *71*(7), 2106–2114.

Lovas, J. (2015). Evidence-Based relaxation therapy: physiological and psychological benefits. *Journal of the Australian Traditional-Medicine Society*, *21*(2), 105.

Lowen, A., & Lowen, L. (2003). *The way to vibrant health: A manual of bioenergetics.* Bioenergetics Press.

Lusebrink, V. B. (1990). *Imagery and visual expression in therapy.* Plenum Press.

Mandel, S. E., Davis, B. A., & Secic, M. (2013). Effects of music therapy and music-assisted relaxation and imagery on health-related outcomes in diabetes education: A feasibility study. *The Diabetes Educator, 39*(4), 568–581.

Mehling, W. E., Wrubel, J., Daubenmier, J. J., Price, C. J., Kerr, C. E., Silow, T., & Stewart, A. L. (2011). Body Awareness: A phenomenological inquiry into the common ground of mind-body therapies. *Philosophy, Ethics, and Humanities in Medicine, 6*, 1–12.

Morton, K., & Cescato, M. (2000). The efficacy of relaxation training with Year 12 students. *Australian Journal of Guidance* and *Counselling, 10*(1), 133–144.

Nurlela, N., & Jannati, Z. (2019). Relaxation technique within group counseling to reduce student's anxiety on facing exam. *Islamic Guidance and Counseling Journal, 2*(1), 33–39.

Ogden, P., & Fisher, J. (2015). *Sensorimotor psychotherapy: Interventions for trauma and attachment.* W.W. Norton & Co.

Ost, L. G. (1987). Applied relaxation: Description of a coping technique and review of controlled studies. *Behaviour Research and Therapy, 25*(5), 397–409.

Pindus, D. M., Lloyd, K. M., Ligeza, T. S., Askow, A., McKenna, C., Bashir, N., & Hillman, C. H. (2025). Interrupting sitting with moderate-intensity physical activity breaks improves cognitive processing speed in adults with overweight and obesity: Findings from the SITLess pilot randomized crossover trial. *International Journal of Psychophysiology, 192*, 112519.

Rosenberg, M. S., Wilson, R., Maheady, L., & Sindelar, P. T. (1997). *Educating students with behavior disorders* (2nd ed.). Allyn & Bacon.

Tsakiris, M., Schütz-Bosbach, S., & Gallagher, S. (2007). On agency and body-ownership: Phenomenological and neurocognitive reflections. *Consciousness and Cognition, 16*(3), 645–660.

Vasu, D. T., Nordin, N. A. M., Xu, S. X., Ghazali, S. E., & Zarim, S. N. A. (2020). Feasibility and outcomes of autogenic relaxation training in addition to usual physiotherapy for stroke survivors. A pilot study. *Malaysian Journal of Public Health Medicine, 20*(3), 134–139.

7 Emotional Integration

Using Emotion-Focused Processes

Emotional Regulation

Moving towards emotional balance, or regulation, of emotions is a natural direction in the psyche, just as in the body there are systems aiming to establish physiological homeostasis. Just as the body rarely stays long in equilibrium (e.g., we are energised, tired, hungry, satiated), so emotions come and go almost constantly, sometimes swinging from pleasant to unpleasant and back again. Of course, when there are unresolved emotions, regulation, return to a balanced state, may be delayed. Emotion regulation is critical both in initiating, motivating and organising adaptive behaviour, and in preventing stressful levels of negative emotions and maladaptive behaviour (Cicchetti et al., 1995). This chapter explores ways to support clients to resolve difficult emotions and increase their ability to regulate emotional expression.

As discussed earlier, within a person-centred approach, the issues, topics, feelings and timing for emotional resolution proceed logically, even if the logic is not clear to the client or the counsellor. Therapy that guides clients through difficult emotions to resolution may involve an initial focus on accessing emotions and somatic experience. In emotion-focused stages of therapy, completing unfinished business, accessing and acknowledging unresolved or incomplete emotions can empower creative, rational choice, productive action and enhanced ability to focus on learning tasks.

Within therapy, adults and children engage in and experience emotional processes in different ways. In general, adults are more willing and able to connect internally, whereas young people focus on survival and establishing a place in the world. Emotion-focused processes may therefore be brief and engaged with just enough to enable moving on.

Why Process Emotional Stress?

During maturation, emotional development precedes most forms of cognitive development (Greenberg, 2006). This means that children experience emotions and react to them before they can articulate their experience or understand it. Young clients are often referred to counselling due to acting-out.

DOI: 10.4324/9781003671879-7

Acting-out is often fuelled by, and eventually adds to, emotional stress. Acting-out could be viewed as (1) an attempt of the psyche to reduce stress, (2) a symptom of the need for resolution. However, acting-out occurs in the wrong place, at the wrong time, unfairly onto others, without therapeutic support or integration. Acting-out behaviours do not lead to resolution or to productive action steps. They do not help the young person connect with underlying primary emotions, such as hurt or fear, and definitely do not lead to approval, support and self-esteem. Without dealing with the emotions that drive acting-out, there is reduced opportunity to reconnect with a positive sense of self.

Emotions need to move. If feelings are simply managed, controlled, or quarantined, with no safe expression or resolution, they remain active and can jeopardise self-efficacy. Suppressed emotion can be acted out destructively through direct and indirect aggression. Sometimes a young client has learned to lock in and disconnect from difficult feelings. This can lead to withdrawal, and over the long term can lead to psychological and health concerns.

Allowing feelings to be felt and safely expressed promotes a state of mental wellbeing, and this may need the framework of an emotion-focused ET activity. Restriction on the expression of feelings can result in a sense of heaviness, irritability, tiredness, depression or a lack of enthusiasm. Ultimately, inhibited emotional expression contributes to behavioural challenges. When supporting young clients in a way that deliberately makes space for emotions, it is first necessary to establish a positive relationship that has a high degree of trust from both therapist and client. Muscular contraction and reduction of breath are automatically employed to contain emotions. After establishing trust, therapeutic work may begin with relaxing or freeing up the body and opening breath.

Some theorists (e.g., Greenberg [2002] writing about Emotion-focused Therapy) distinguish between primary emotion and secondary emotion. Secondary emotion can be a reaction to the primary emotion; e.g., anger can be a reaction to being hurt or afraid. Ideally, for long-term therapeutic benefit, it is valuable to experience and process the primary emotion. It can be helpful to support clients to "track back" to the primary feeling, sometimes through layers of emotion. Additionally, anger and frustration can also be reactions to suppression of positive qualities and states, such as excitement, individuality, creativity or simply being energetic.

In living with contained emotions, feelings of strength and vitality are also held back. Personal authority, aliveness, assertiveness and a positive sense of self diminish when emotion has no outlet. The result can be low self-esteem.

Intrapersonal Sources of Challenging Behaviours

In emotionally stressful situations, feelings that are too strong for a young person to deal with, or that are not accepted by others, or that are not safe to express, may be pushed out of awareness. A person may "forget" the feelings and even the stressful situation. They can move to implicit memory. This automatic survival or self-protection process of repression was first identified by Freud and described in 1915. Repression offers an essential and common emotional defence or survival mechanism.

Despite being forgotten, these stressful feelings remain active forces and influence the hormonal system, generate contraction in the muscular system, in the neural circuits, the nervous system as a whole and automatic constriction in the respiratory system. Clearly, an effective therapeutic response is multi-modal, aiming to gently soften these holding systems. Tension generated by the effort of containing feelings and the inclination to express them significantly increases emotional stress. Unfinished business and associated feelings exert more influence on behaviour than intentional plans, and then begin to shape self-image and character.

Reactions from others to emotional expression, throughout the developmental years, mean emotional distress is often controlled, diverted, reasoned away, modified, soothed and calmed, squashed or ignored. Consequences of suppression of emotion include depression, addiction, illness and violence (Payne, 1985). In general, unexpressed, unresolved feelings have a disruptive influence on behaviour, learning and relating. They contribute to psychosomatic symptoms and health issues. So, can we provide more opportunities within counselling for the unresolved emotional life to emerge and be worked through?

Interpersonal Support through Applying ET

Acknowledging, validating and accepting children's emotional life allows both natural, regular expression and promotes the capacity to experience and process emotions in a healthy way. However, since this is not widely welcomed in many settings, a young person may have developed habitual constriction; habits that include fear of approaching difficult emotions. A common concern is that addressing emotion within sessions may lead to increased levels of acting-out at home and school. There are very significant and clear differences between acting-out difficult feelings (where behaviour is disruptive and unfair) and therapeutic processing within a safe therapeutic relationship.

Therapeutic processing of difficult emotions needs to take place in a contained, safe, private setting, under the guidance of an accepting and qualified counsellor. Emotion-focused processes with ET allow the client choice of expressive modalities, choice of emotional depth or experiencing. This choice, and the ET invitational way of relating, ensures minimum risk of overwhelm. Emotion-focused processes take place through the body, leading to relaxation and providing space for cognitive re-appraisal. Most importantly, the processes are followed by integration activities that allow access to more positive emotions, including those evoked by therapist acceptance. This activates greater approval from self and others.

The ET emotion-focused activity examples in this book can provide a range of safe structured therapeutic activities for accessing, identifying and symbolising emotion; for releasing, completing, integrating and reflecting on emotional experiences, as well as contributing to more objective planning of new strategies. Young people can learn to prefer therapeutic release over acting-out and even use emotion processing activities as self-support.

Psychological and Emotional Integration

While each client is unique, with their own pathway through therapy, our clinical observations from a combined 70 years have identified six typical steps or stages in the transformational process. The first step, typical of most therapy, is supporting the client to enhance their awareness or recognition of their current state, their somatic signals, their automatic thoughts and primarily their feelings and reactions.

Where a client has learned to ignore or suppress unfinished business, hurts, disappointments, the second step brings the challenge to relax efforts to ignore or avoid those experiences. There may be a need for a clear rationale for relaxing defensiveness. Often closely associated with this is the third step of relaxing efforts to understand, to let go of protective cognitive mechanisms or tendencies to focus on finding reasons for experience, rather than experiencing. Covering early hurts and disappointments with adult information may have been a useful protective mechanism; however, in many cases, it can result in self-blaming. Participation in a warm and empathic therapeutic relationship, with gentle encouragement to stay internally focused, may be essential to enable readiness to make contact with self.

The fourth step invites the client to allow experience and expression of layers of emotions. While there is no routine pattern, these layers may initially present for many clients as frustration, anger, resentment or even as a drive towards revenge-seeking. Greenberg would call this a secondary layer of emotion. When the client is able to experience and express their reactions there may be a natural movement to make contact with the background or primary feelings. Feelings of hurt or disappointment, of not being loved enough, or listened to, or held, respected, or safe, may arise, sometimes unexpectedly. For some, there may even be a further underlying layer of more vulnerable feelings related to early survival fears.

A fifth step in the therapeutic process emerges when a client is supported to stay with – and move through – difficult feelings, to arrive at an underlying positive, quiet state. While in steps three and four there is a focus on supporting direct emotional experience, in this calmer fifth step there is a focus on a more centred connection with self. Reflection and understanding are invited to lead to sustainable problem-solving, formulating appropriate aims and strategies.

Therapeutic presence and care provide the sixth step, where a "corrective experience" of acceptance supports client self-acceptance and interest in self-care, creativity and the overall development of resilience.

What Are Emotion-Focused Processes?

Within the therapeutic setting, contact with powerful emotion contributes "to metamorphoses of the self", and becomes the central agent responsible for therapeutic change (Fosha, 2000). Fosha found that "core affective states" contain powerful adaptive forces and processes with a heightened therapeutic potential capable of accelerating therapeutic change. These adaptive forces emerge naturally when a child is safe and free to play (Lowenfeld, 1935).

Processing difficult or unresolved feelings with therapeutic activities can lead to emotional regulation. Processing facilitates the release of reactivity, completing unfinished business, allowing a natural process of emotional connection – or exposure – and expression to take place. The main aim is to support an internal encounter with incomplete emotions and reactions from the present and the past.

Emotion-focused processes usually take place in three basic stages:

1. Preparation, including discussion of current concerns, especially any emotional distress or reactivity;
2. Processing, via strategies to support connecting with emotions, and their activating situations, expression and release;
3. Integration, understanding and closure.

Emotion-focused processes offer clients an opportunity to cross thresholds from ignoring to talking about a difficult event, to exploring the experience and resolution. Structurally, these processes may involve steps that surrender rational containment, increase somatic awareness and reconnection with emotion, safe expression, then resolution, leading to clearer self-understanding. Effectiveness is enhanced by increasing self-awareness and encouraging some deeper breaths and movement where possible. Processing can lead to closure and supports the formulation of new direction, aims and strategies. Fosha (2000) describes an energetic outcome from processing deep emotion: Access to new resources and renewed energy. This leads to what she terms "adaptive action tendencies", and the ability to adapt is at the heart of developing resilience.

Outcomes from Emotion-Focused Processes

This summary of outcomes is based on the literature, the authors' clinical observations, and anecdotal reports from our clients and supervisees. There are three main areas of outcomes: Emotional, cognitive and relational. Importantly, there are some contra-indications that need to be considered (see page 179). Adjustment symptoms may also be evident at times for some clients.

When a client works through emotion-laden distress, changes observed include: Calmer mood, less aggression, less anxiety, increased self-assurance and assertiveness (Pearson, 2003); sense of freedom, lightness and balance

(Pearson & Wilson, 2008); emotional strength and reconnection with a stable sense of self, resourcefulness and creativity; increased sense of self-acceptance; more hopeful view of the future (Pearson & Wilson, 2001); confidence (Pearson, 2006) aliveness and meaning (Fosha, 2000). Additionally, ET processes also support heightened professional satisfaction in practitioners (Holian, 2001; O'Brien & Burnett, 2000; Pearson, 2003; Tereba, 1999).

Therapeutic outcomes often include capacity to self-regulate, reduction in aggressive behaviour and decreased anxiousness. There can be a notable reduction in reactive behaviours, and for some clients, a corresponding increase in the ability to be appropriately assertive. Some clients display an increased sense of confidence, strength, resourcefulness and creativity, along with greater awareness of emotions in general.

As noted by Greenberg (2004), some clients experience more positive emotional states with an increased sense of self-acceptance. There is often a decrease in automatic negative thoughts and less self-criticism. Many young clients quickly develop a more hopeful view of the future and are able to draw on their inner-life skills. After anger-focused processes, there can be a sense of renewed energy, with a decrease in self-blaming and more self-compassion. After experiencing grief, most clients display initial tiredness, followed by refreshed energy; however, they can temporarily feel more vulnerable.

Improved attention spans and renewed interest in learning are the most recognisable cognitive outcomes. Along with this, an increased capacity for creative problem-solving and openness to reflect on self, along with awareness of the "other" (i.e., mentalising ability), is enhanced. Relational or social outcomes include an improved capacity to relate positively, with less reactivity or hidden agenda. Willingness to cooperate and make psychologically healthier choices with positive action tendencies can parallel a more hopeful worldview.

It is normal to note some adjustment symptoms. These may relate to external influences and the relational re-adjustment of significant others. For example, while now more in touch with, and expressive of, feelings, this may not be welcomed by a client's immediate social or familial network. Adolescents in particular may feel uncomfortable with a new sense of openness and vulnerability after sessions. It is vital to discuss these temporary possibilities with clients and explain them to families in a context of change.

Reducing the Effects of Emotional Distress

Our human body produces both physiological and behavioural responses to perceived stressors. The body attempts to overcome the perceived threat of stress and protect itself. Protection involves responses of the endocrine system, the autonomic nervous system and the immune system (Dhabhar, 2013; McEwen, 2007). In other words, adverse life experiences lead to changes in the chemistry and physiology of the body.

These responses may, however, lead to disturbances of mental, emotional and behavioural functioning over the long term. There is considerable evidence that the body responds to stress through increases in the levels of hormones, such as adrenaline, norepinephrine and cortisol. Chronic cortisol elevation can have detrimental effects on health: It increases the risk of atherosclerosis and heart disease, and can lead to health challenges in older age; it may contribute to diabetes and to depression; it can also impede the person's immune function (Kadzikowska-Wrzosek, 2012).

Depending on their level of resilience, clients are affected by emotional distress – sometimes more or less. Emotional stress can be a by-product of living in, trying to defend against threats in a negative environment; from coping which involves holding back feelings from expression, and from efforts to overcome the impact of the strong feelings of others. Added to this are internal attempts not to acknowledge emotional distress, to create distance from it.

Long-term emotional distress can show up in behavioural difficulties such as acting-out or withdrawal. Long-term emotional distress contributes to emotional difficulties (e.g., anxiety and depression), cognitive impairment and learning problems, and to chronic physical tension, weaker blood circulation and related immune system weaknesses, as well as a decrease in general health. Sufficient evidence exists that highlights the detrimental effect of stressful life events on both physical and mental health (Kadzikowska-Wrzosek, 2012).

ET activities support developing self-regulation for young people, so as to minimise the risk of harmful effects of stressful situations. Our clinical observations over many years suggest that short-term and long-term emotional stress can contribute to and cause: Headaches and stomach aches, body pains – especially chest and back, mouth ulcers, muscle cramps, skin problems, bladder problems, nausea and digestive upsets, nightmares and eating difficulties. These symptoms have been identified in the literature for some time as potentially having their origin in stress (e.g., Greene & Walker, 1997; Kelly et al., 2010). Several symptoms are commonly reported as co-existing, and one or two (or more) of the symptoms may indicate that having time and safety to process emotional stress can be important for the reduction in emotional overwhelm.

Childhood Scripts and Reactive Behaviour

The three main influences in the development of the psyche are: Biographical experiences since birth (scripts, schemas, internal working models, core beliefs); perinatal experiences (around birth), considered by many as the first lessons about life; and transpersonal (metaphysical or spiritual). However, counsellors mainly focus on dealing with the aftermath of biographical events, the way these generate beliefs, emotional patterns and behaviours. An approach, therefore, that incorporates psychodynamic understanding is recommended.

Childhood scripts – or "injunctions" or "emotional schemas" – are conditioned patterns of belief, emotion and behaviour. These schemas may be out of awareness, having formed "blue-prints" or prototypes from our earliest times. Bowlby (1988) used the term "internal working models". These models, or scripts, are learned, programmed emotional codes that can incline us to habitually react to certain situations in the same way over time. They set in place beliefs about self and the world. These scripts can be positive or negative. It is the power of negative scripts that most needs to be explored in therapy, and that often underlie challenging feelings and behaviours.

A script has emotional, cognitive and behavioural components: Suppressed feelings connected with emotional pain; negative or limiting beliefs about self; along with behaviour patterns that contribute to defending against emotional pain. When scripts are activated by a current incident, previous hurts, disappointments, resentments from the past are activated at the same time. This double reaction may be evident in an "over-the-top" way when reactions seem out of proportion.

Positive life experiences, early security and fulfilment, that contribute to building resilience do not require therapeutic attention. However, it can be useful to bring these to the forefront and reinforce them through symbolising strengths and resilience.

Young clients with ongoing challenges may benefit from working through experiences that drive reactivity. Not feeling good enough, not feeling loved or valued, held or validated, the legacy of not feeling lovable generates undercurrents of resentment. Anger and resentment are often the unexpressed reaction to feeling hurt. Counselling can support feeling safe enough to make contact with underlying vulnerabilities. There can be a need to reduce the automatic nature of reactions. This entails drawing awareness to emotions, allowing some expression of them, gaining understanding of them, and bringing integration in a way that reduces reactive impulses.

How counsellors respond to and handle reports of young clients' acting-out, or acting-out events within a therapeutic space, can contribute to reducing or reinforcing a client's negative beliefs about self. A client-focused approach offers ideal conditions to reduce the negative influences of a client's scripts. Judgement is replaced with acceptance. A corrective experience is provided through positive emotion within a therapeutic alliance, and from a safe, supported experience of acknowledging, expressing and releasing unprocessed emotion.

Some typical negative scripts, beliefs or self-talk that challenge clients include:

- *I'm not good enough … to be loved/respected/safe/held.*
- *I'm not clever enough …*
- *I am not attractive*
- *No one really likes me/I'm not wanted*
- *I will miss out*
- *It is not safe here/not safe to speak out*
- *How I am is not OK.*

Supporting Emotion-Focused Processes

Principles of Emotional Transformation

Creation of a sense of safety in the therapeutic relationship is always the first task. When safety is experienced, clients are more willing to be aware of emotions or open to feeling vulnerable. ET aims to create a rationale for clients to be willing to move past experiential avoidance and tolerate emotion-laden experiences in therapy.

A prelude to offering activities that have the potential to bring forward emotional reactivity is establishing clear boundaries. These include behavioural boundaries where it is clear that no acting-out will inflict injury to self, others or surroundings. Boundaries are clear between therapeutic processes that support expression and acting-out beyond the consulting room. Time boundaries and clear indicators of time remaining are offered by the counsellor.

Support Guidelines

Young clients often need to move towards experiencing their core concerns slowly and indirectly. They may not be able to clearly recall or be willing to speak about difficult or traumatic events. In many cases, symbolic, nonverbal expression offers a safe alternative; for example, expressing emotion through art, through stories using miniatures or through movement or animal role-play.

Do not rush the process, follow the client's timing, allow time pauses, encourage the client to give themselves time to reflect and feel, free from pressure to come up with explanations. Allow times of silence, even if these seem uncomfortable. Pause time helps the client make contact with emotion and reflect on their experiences. Encourage the client to see if there are any impulses, movements or actions that would naturally accompany their process.

From an ET perspective, change is seen as occurring by helping people experience and understand their emotions through the six steps of (1) awareness, (2) expression, (3) integration, (4) reflection, (5) transformation in an environment offering (6) corrective experiences of an empathically attuned therapeutic relationship. It can be tempting to bypass the crucial second step of expression if we ourselves are not comfortable with dealing with strong emotion. ET provides many practical activities to support connection with emotion and its expression. While we recognise these six main steps in dealing with emotion, the process is not linear, and stages are likely to overlap.

1. Awareness: After establishing some rapport, when the client is ready, guide their focus to increase awareness of emotion. Support clients to accept, tolerate, stay with, then externalise or symbolise emotions. This can be supported through body focus, followed by expression with words, miniatures and colours, lines and shapes. Support to extend this emotional literacy will enhance clients' abilities to communicate about emotion.

2. Emotional expression: Support clients to express emotions. Expression may be direct and verbal, or indirect, expressed symbolically, through movement games, emotional release games, role-play, bioenergetics, as well as through process art and writing.

   Clients can be supported to experiment with colours, lines, shapes that represent their feelings, moods and reactions. Clients can be encouraged to draw continuously (process art) until a difficult feeling seems discharged. One way to evoke this expression is to use an imaginary encounter, similar to the Gestalt two-chair process. Imagining an encounter with the source of reactions will support connection with, and expression of, negative emotional reactivity. Young clients can be empowered to express through imagining the "other" as smaller (see "The Dot on the Wall" page 190). The "other" in the imagined encounter can also be represented via a sketch or a selection of miniatures. Alternatively, clients can imagine self as growing bigger and stronger in order to reduce the perceived hierarchy of age and size, (as in "Finding my Animal Sounds", see page 189).
3. Integration and emotional regulation: Emotional integration can be enhanced through the provision of a safe, calming, validating and empathic environment, wherein the client can develop distress tolerance skills. These skills may include: identifying and labelling emotions, allowing and tolerating difficult emotions, increasing positive emotions, self-soothing and being able to identify and understand future activating encounters. Simple forms of somatic mindfulness for grounding, that combine breath awareness, relaxation and self-accepting dialogue may be very helpful here (see pages from 210 to 217).
4. Reflection: The fourth stage involves reflection or making sense of the therapeutic experience. Invite the client to reflect on their emotional experience, to find what information the experience holds, what they can discover from it, bringing order out of confusion and chaos. This discussion leads to further self-understanding and revised perspectives on self, others and the world. Reflection contributes to the development of increased sensitivity that can alert the young person to future times when emotion processing might be useful.
5. Emotional transformation: When difficult emotions have been expressed and understood, there is usually a resultant positive state. Greenberg (2015) describes transforming challenging emotions such as fear, shame, the sadness of being abandoned or alone, with other adaptive emotions. Help young clients take time to tune into emerging positive states, to embody calm and balance. Their experiences of emotional transformation can enhance willingness to engage in therapy and adopt self-management abilities.
6. Corrective emotional experience: While this should, ideally, be part of an overall person-centred counselling experience, a priority at this stage is that the counsellor provides a sense of presence to the client's new,

sometimes vulnerable, state. The ongoing relationship with a mindful and caring counsellor can provide a new lived experience that transforms previous patterns of negativity. Therapists provide a corrective relational experience. Additionally, positive feedback on the client's engagement in therapy can consolidate a "success experience".

Questions to consider when preparing to support an emotion-focused activity:

- *Has there been sufficient time and engagement to build a level of trust and rapport with the client?*
- *Has there been time to be curious about the client, to understand their emotional needs, their vulnerability and resilience?*
- *Has a plan of possible activities been considered to provide choice for the client?*
- *Have the activities been worked with or experienced personally?*
- *Are resources and equipment prepared?*
- *Does the consulting room have a level of visual and auditory privacy?*
- *Will it be possible to maintain confidentiality for written, spoken or drawn expressions?*
- *Is the workspace ordered, with positive and respectful preparation?*
- *Are there large cushions to sit on, jump on, or even lash out at if needed?*
- *Is there a range of drawing paper and crayons for written, visual and symbolic expression?*
- *Are there miniatures available as a focus for creating an imaginary encounter?*
- *Are tissues within reach?*

Ways to Work through Difficult Emotion: A Summary

Body focus: Locating feelings on a body outline
Bioenergetic exercises
Physical and energetic release games
Writing activities:

- process writing
- imaginary letters
- sentence starters
- reflective writing – with guiding questions
- completion writing – summaries

Visual art:

- process drawing, drawing feelings, emotional release drawing
- drawing to emotionally orientated music
- sculpting feelings with clay
- completion mandalas

Emotion-focused Processes

- activities that focus clients directly on their feelings
- may use an imaginary encounter

Working with music:

- draw to emotionally evocative music
- client selects music to correspond to a range of feelings (also develops emotional literacy)
- movement (or dance) to emotionally evocative music
- express feelings using percussion instruments.

Skills for Facilitation

Flow with the Client: While ET provides many activities that lead a client towards experience, remember to follow their process, trust the logic of their readiness to participate, or not. Stay open to indications from the client about what needs to happen next.

Minimum Verbal Direction: Offer a structure with steps and stages and lots of flexibility. Avoid giving advice, offering re-frames, solutions or imposing viewpoints during emotional exploration. Don't distract the client from direct emotional and somatic awareness.

Do Not Impose Your Interpretations onto the Client: While remaining present and assessing the client's emotional state, don't try to convey your perceptions. Engage the client in self-exploration through the use of very open, invitational, reflection-activating questions, based on your observations, in order to help the client deepen self-connection and arrive at their own understanding.

Mirror: Occasionally reflect back some of the client's key words, phrases and feelings. Sometimes it can be helpful to invite the client to repeat key phrases; this aids self-connection.

Support Emotional Experiencing and Expression: Encourage clients to increase awareness of and expression of their emotions. Try not to manage their feelings. Give permission, encouragement and time for expression, in their own way, and to the degree they are comfortable with.

Be Aware of Self and Relax: Practice divided attention: Attention on both self and the client leads to therapeutic presence. Your mindful presence involves regularly returning to self-awareness, taking steady full breaths, opening and relaxing your posture and generally practising self-awareness. Note any hopes, expectations or agendas that may arise and may need to be dealt with in supervision.

Welcome Your "Creative Doubt" and Open to Informed Intuition: In ET it is normal to be unsure of exactly what to do or say next. Creative doubt is a calm state of not-knowing and waiting for clues on how to proceed. Relax with not-knowing, befriend this state, open to perception, and allow some silence. Informed intuition includes receiving clues from the client; noticing your internal impressions, recalling theoretical frameworks; and an array of skills.

Creating a Safe Environment

As mentioned, therapeutic effectiveness can be enhanced when sufficient trust and rapport develop. The timing for offering emotion-focused processes will depend on:

- a client's sense of safety
- when a client's self-awareness has developed
- when activities are provided to externalise reactions, and
- when time and methods for integration are supplied.

In summary, clients need structure, privacy, trust and integration opportunities to support effective outcomes.

The physical environment contributes to enabling successful emotion-focused outcomes. If possible, offer soft natural light to support relaxation. Some quiet background music can support a client's feeling of privacy and readiness to focus internally. Energetic, strong music can support the expression of emotion; gentle music can assist contact with grief or vulnerability, and calm music with a slow beat can support integration.

There are many components of an emotionally supportive work space (See Pearson & Wilson, 2012). A sound-proof, private room with space to move about if needed is ideal. Carpet, mats or soft floor covering are recommended. Overall, the room should feel safe and comfortable to the client, being ordered, clean, and with a sense of beauty. Order and attractive impressions help to make a space psychologically safe for clients and convey a message of respect.

Specific equipment will include tissues, art-making materials, paper to rip, beeswax or clay or plasticine for moulding shapes and symbols, writing materials, and it can be ideal to provide stickers for those concerned about their artistic skills. It is ideal if a collection of miniatures is available, as well as recorded music equipment – and access to a broad selection of music styles. Music-making instruments such as drums, percussion instruments, and possibly a keyboard can expand client options for expression.

Integration after Emotion-Focused Processes

Emotion-focused activities should only be offered when there is sufficient time for integration and closure, time for reflection and discussion, time for body and mind to readjust after the process. Integration is Step 4 of the ET 5-Stage Model, where grounding and reflection are encouraged. The client is encouraged to understand their experiences in the session and to relax. The integration stage links right hemisphere brain experience with left hemisphere reflection, naming, description and time-sequencing. Stimulation of the left hemisphere can result in positive awareness and elevated optimistic motivation (Stien & Kendall, 2014). Integration using calming, verbal and non-verbal reflective activities, and/or silent creative expression time, for example with mandala creation, and the sharing of the experience with a "trusted guide", consolidates experience.

The integration stage supports a client to interpret their experience, and begin to view their life from a broader perspective. In this calmer space, they can begin to consider self-care, identify where support might be needed, and envision new directions. The most commonly used integration activity is discussion, to:

- invite a client to reflect on the impact of the activity,
- assess any further support that would be useful,
- focus on client's hopes and projects for the future,
- develop new strategies and practical steps,
- consider new ways to manage self and use energy positively and productively.

Therapeutic writing with a private journal can also evoke cognitive review when a client may not wish to disclose their experiences. Therapeutic writing activities may include non-directed spontaneous writing, invitations to respond to set questions, and the use of sentence starters (see more on p. 107 to 110).

Relaxation and visualisation activities can also support calming and closure; however, especially for younger children, rhythmic movement may be what they prefer. Movement activities may best suit clients who feel safe, energised or triumphant after an emotion-focused activity, for example, a short informal walk around the consulting room, structured movement such as bioenergetic exercises, and free play with large cushions, for example, jumping or rolling over them.

Contraindications and Providing Safety

There are two main types of emotion-focused processes used in ET:

1. those that allow some spontaneous contact with and expression of emotional stress, where the counsellor follows and supports the client's direction; and

2. those that are designed to activate connection with the expression of emotions.

This second type of process deals with a range of active emotions that may be out of a client's immediate awareness. In these cases, the activity structure may more definitely invite the client into the process. It is always ideal to seek clinical supervision if there is any doubt about client readiness or suitability for emotion-focused work.

Do not use processes that lead a client towards activation of issues if: There is insufficient trust established; if a client has no prior experience with you; if you do not know the client well enough to make a clear assessment; if there is no support or understanding of therapy from carers; if there is a clash of counsellor and carer paradigms, (e.g., about empowerment or the value of emotional awareness) or if the client doesn't want to do it. Be concerned if there are tight time limits that could curtail integration and closure.

If client – or counsellor – has limited or no framework or rationale for emotion-focused activities, work in a more indirect symbolic way. If the client has in the past shown a consistent lack of behavioural boundaries when emotions are active, avoid both types of processes. If there is uncertainty about medications – e.g., sedatives, anti-depressants, ADHD medications, avoid intentional activation of emotion. And if a client has a history of psychiatric treatment that could suggest some confusion about boundaries and internal symbolic processes and acting-out, avoid the second more directed type of process.

Finally, if you are not comfortable with emotion-focused work, or if your intuition/gut feeling is against using expressive processes, avoid them, even if reasons are not clear. In general, do not use an activity you have not explored personally, or for which you have no appropriate training.

Emotional Literacy and Inner-Life Skills

Participation in ET sessions can have a positive impact on discovery, processing and learning about emotions. Engaging in the ET activities can develop emotional literacy (EL) skills, which in turn contribute to client resilience. This section introduces emotional literacy and describes what we call "Inner-Life skills" for self-management that can be developed through participation in activity-based ET sessions. This "educational" contribution of ET assists clients to gain understanding of their internal processes, as well as deepen their engagement in therapy and resilience in daily life.

The term "emotional literacy" has been defined as "our ability to recognise, manage, comprehend and suitably communicate our emotions and to understand how they shape our actions and relationships and influence our thinking" (Spendlove, 2008, p. 4).

A sense of meaning and purpose is derived as much from feeling as from understanding. Emotions are directly connected with motivation and cognitive development (Sharp, 2001). Sharp describes how dealing with emotions can help to develop improved relationship skills and a sense of psychological and mental wellbeing. Furthermore, emotionally developed young people have been found to be better equipped to live with difference (Sharp, 2001).

We have identified three main types of inner-life skills (ILS) developed when clients use ET: Intrapersonal, interpersonal and transpersonal. Together they correlate with three intelligences, named by Gardner (2006) as intrapersonal intelligence (others call this emotional intelligence), interpersonal intelligence (others call this social intelligence), and a proposed metaphysical or existential intelligence (named by some authors as spiritual intelligence).

Intrapersonal Inner-Life Skills

A natural ability with the intrapersonal intelligence brings enjoyment and learning through self-reflection; through metacognition and through working alone; as well as awareness of inner spiritual realities (Armstrong, 1994). There are five categories of intrapersonal ILS.

1. **Self-Awareness and Self-Knowledge**: These include the ability with somatic awareness, emotional awareness, awareness of beliefs about self – both positive and negative, awareness of energy and impulses – for example, the flow or stasis of energy, the build-up and activation of impulses, as well as ability with self-care – for example, through using relaxation, mindfulness and meditation, imagery and symbol.
2. **Self-Understanding and Self-Acceptance**: The skills of self-understanding and self-acceptance include awareness of, and relative freedom from, self-criticism or automatic negative thoughts. The skill of recognising the automatic process of self-criticism – rather than believing that negative self-talk is fact – is an essential step. The ability to reflect on behaviour and beliefs – and perhaps in time, the sources of them – is a hoped-for direction in therapy. A willingness to explore symbolic imagery in metaphor, dreams, fantasies, artwork and symbol work is one that can develop over time for clients engaged in ET. Developing personal mythology – recognising ongoing meaningful personal themes – metaphors and symbols, or totems, could be seen as a skill in greater understanding of self. The ability to notice intuition, hunches, gut feelings and internal guidance can develop as clients become comfortable with self-awareness.
3. **Emotional Literacy**: While all the inner-life skills could be seen as components of, or contributors to, emotional literacy, there are components of EL that quite specifically deal with emotion. The ability to express emotion and communicate about feelings can be developed, both within therapy and ideally as a way of living that improves social skills and reduces acting-out. Initially, identifying and naming emotions forms a foundation for EL. Gradually using more complex symbols other than words

to identify, process and communicate emotion can be encouraged, for example, expression through line, colour, shape and image; then through speech and the written word, as well as expression through the body.

4. **Managed Emotional and Physical Release**: Ideally, within therapy, clients are supported to work through difficult emotions. Sometimes, simple and safe ways for venting can be taught as a management tool. For example, the use of bioenergetics, movement and expressive games and role-play.

5. **Self-direction and Motivation**: These skills can best be developed after initial experiences with ET. The ability to self-evaluate, to use reflection and visualisation develops later in therapy. Development of the skills of discerning inner wisdom or a sense of what is right and wrong or what is most needed in a moment can grow over time through ET. Focus on Step 5 of our 5-Stage Model: The Way Forward, increases a client's ability to determine creative use of energy and formulate productive strategies to deal with problems. Gentle questioning from an empathic counsellor can bring forward skills in recognising hopes, dreams and directions for the future. Having direction, hope and focus for the future is an ideal outcome.

Interpersonal Inner-Life Skills

These support and use interpersonal intelligence and are particularly well learned and consolidated within a group context. Someone with a natural ability in this domain learns and operates one-to-one through group relationships and communication. The two categories within interpersonal ILS are relationships to others and support of others. These skills are more obviously developed within groupwork.

Relationship to Others: Developing empathy, being able to perceive others' moods and states is a valuable inner-life skill. The skill of understanding the dynamics of a group or classroom or family, and being able to adjust to or anticipate these dynamics may contribute to resilience. Being able to recognise and deal with the negative reactions of others, and maintain a sense of self in the face of pressure, is a skill that evolves within emotion-focused ET. Being able to visualise and consider others' needs may be the ILS that parents would most like support to develop in their offspring. Modelling respect, empathy, interest and sensitivity through person-centred practice may help with this.

Support of Others: The skill of being an emotional support for another is welcomed by many young people. Adolescent clients thrive in well-run groupwork when they feel these skills expand their repertoire for relating effectively. In groupwork, there are, for example, opportunities to teach and practice active listening. Emotional and empathic support experiences, with others who may be feeling vulnerable, are highly growth-promoting.

Transpersonal Inner-Life Skills

These utilise an existential intelligence. We are accepting that this cluster of cognitive abilities exists, although Gardner makes it clear that according to his scientific data it cannot be confirmed. Existential intelligence has been described as exploring the nature of existence and is explicitly concerned with spiritual or religious matters (Armstrong, 1994).

Within transpersonal inner-life skills, the central category could be described as sensitivity and capacity to reflect on deep questions about existence, the meaning of life, why we exist, and how we get here? Simmons (2006) argues for the importance of providing means for young people to reflect on existential issues. Kalff (2003) observed that many of her adolescent clients undertaking psychotherapy via Sandplay Therapy developed an interest in existence and shared with her their metaphysical questions. We have similar observations from sessions with clients of all ages. Responding to client interest, meeting their need to know or question through providing the means for articulating the questioning process symbolically builds this skill.

PRACTICAL EMOTION-FOCUSED ACTIVITIES

Activity 7.1 Emotional Literacy Development: *Times of Feeling Good and Not so Good*

Suggested Age Range: From eight to nine years.
Materials: An A3 sheet of paper, crayons, access to the Feeling Words and Shapes Lists (Appendix B – pp. 252–254).
Preparation: Divide an A3 size sheet of paper into three sections.

Read out the following three imaginary scenes to the client. Complete work with each scene before moving on to the next. For each scene, ask clients to:

1. *Tune in to your response when imagining the scene.*
2. *Note how that feels inside you.*
3. *Find a shape that goes with your response to the scene.*
4. *Look at your crayons. What colour would that shape be?*
5. *Draw the shape in a section of the page.*
6. *Find a few feeling words that also go with your response.*
7. *Write the feeling words inside the shape or beside it.*

Scene 1 – Imagine This:
You are walking home from school. You see a group of older kids you don't know, from another school. They turn and look at you. They seem to be laughing.

Scene 2 – Imagine This:
It is late on Sunday night, during the school term. You know you have not finished your homework. It is too late to do anything about it. You don't want to tell your parents.

Scene 3 – Imagine This:
One of the popular kids at school wants to become your friend. It is someone you like. They hang out with you at the weekend, you have pizza and go to a film. You are popular, you have a new friend. You have a great time.

Discussion
Clients are invited to share:

1. what they drew and wrote
2. how they would feel in each scene
3. any times they have felt like any of these scenes
4. any experiences like this that were important to them.

Activity 7.2 Emotional and Somatic Literacy: *Bad Times/Good Times – What's Going on Inside?*

Suggested Age Range: From eight to nine years. Works well as an activity within group work.

Materials: Worksheet: *Bad Times/Good Times*, coloured pencils or crayons, biro.

Rationale: This activity has been designed to help you get clear on how you feel in your body in different situations. Our body is sending us messages about our feelings and thoughts all the time. The more we learn to listen to it, the more we can make useful decisions and know what we really want; we have more choices.

Instructions

1. *I'm inviting you to spend some time quietly working down the two columns; then you can share what you learned if you wish. You will be free to say as much or as little about yourself as you wish. You can decide if you want to show your page to me or keep it private.*
2. *Talking about these things helps us understand ourselves and be understood better by others.*
3. *Starting with the first column, close your eyes and tune in to your body. See if you can remember how it feels inside when important tests, exams, assignments or lots of homework need doing, during times when things are not so good.*
4. *Draw in the first body outline, using any colours, shapes, lines or shading that somehow go with the feelings in your body at that time.*
   - *Is it the same all through the body, or are there some areas that are different?*
   - *Think back – what it was like in your head, in your middle, your arms and hands, your belly, your legs and feet.*
   - *You can also use words here if you want to.*

5. *Next, circle any words in the lists that come closest to describing how you felt inside then.*
6. *Next imagine you are the weather.*
   - *Think of yourself now as the clouds, the heat or the cold, the wind, the rain, snow, the humidity.*
   - *What sort of day would you be shortly before exams or a test?*
   - *Write a brief description of this.*
7. *Next, think about, then write down on the dotted lines, three words or a phrase that describes your attitude to life at these times.*
   - *For example, would your attitude to life be cool? aggro? don't care? focused? give up? it's great? its hopeless?*
8. *If you can't think of anything, simply move on, then come back and spend more time with it.*
9. *The last activity in the column is to think for a moment and see if you can remember any other events or situations when you feel the same way.*
10. *Brief discussion – Talk about the left-hand side.*
11. *Move on to work down the second column when you are ready. Here you are asked to remember how it feels in your body when you are on holiday and having fun with friends, with lots of free time.*
12. *Continue to work down the second column as you did for the first column.*

Discussion

When you have finished, let's talk about:

- *How did you feel doing this page?*
- *Were there any parts of the page you didn't like?*
- *Can you talk about the feelings in your body that you found?*
- *Did you discover anything about yourself?*
- *What parts of the page seemed most important to you?*
- *Can you say more about the "attitudes to life" section?*
- *Can you think of anyone else who has that attitude?*

Integration

Invite the group to share any thoughts or feelings about the contents of the page.

Give permission to add to the page when others express what they wanted to express. It is OK to be inspired by each other.

Activity 7.3 Emotion-Focused Process: *Dealing with Current Reactions*

Suggested Age Range: From nine years.

Materials: Paper, crayons, pen, miniatures, dots, cushions, tissues, space to move, background music.

Purpose: A process to allow the client to express and reduce reactivity and underlying emotions that affect behaviour.

Step 1: Preparation
Help client identify current reactions, upsets, frustrations or strong feelings – through discussion, reflection or somatic focus, and review of recent events.

Step 2: Processing
Encourage the client to make contact with their feelings through:

- activating the body and emotions with bioenergetics or breathing games
- tuning-in to the body, while taking some deep breaths
- spontaneous drawing of feelings.

Collaborate with the client to identify and externalise the focus of reactivity:

- client imagines the person (or group, or place) that they have been reacting to
- client represents the person or place by:
  - drawing something, e.g., a sketch of their face
  - or selecting miniatures to represent them
  - or focuses on a spot (dot) on the wall that can represent them
  - or imagine them seated in an empty chair
  - or simply imagining that they are present.

While looking at the face (or symbol, or spot), client takes several slow, full, deep breaths.

Ask: *Could you imagine the person is here now? Is there anything you would like to say to them? You can now say anything you need to.*

Give clients time to connect with their feelings and find their own way to express themselves.

The client is encouraged to express their reactions while imagining an encounter with the person/place/group. This expression could be:

- whispered,
- spoken aloud,
- shouted,
- written – in words, or even a secret sign language,
- through process drawing (see page 92), with or without words,
- through the use of drums or percussion instruments.

Encourage any somatic expression through moving the body.

- stand up
- hand or arm movements
- move the whole body?

Suggest the client expresses how the situation made them feel.

- *Tell "them" about you.*
- Could you begin: *I felt …*

Encourage some deep breaths and give permission for expressing emotions freely.

Invite the client to articulate what they wanted around the situation (or from the person):

- *Can you say what you really wanted, or did not want?*

Client stands up and is invited to stretch and shake a little.

- *Is there anything more that you want to say?*

Step 3: Integration

After expression, encourage a few minutes of quiet time for self-focus. Invite them to be aware of any sensations, moods or thoughts.

The client is invited to:

- Create an image that shows how they feel now
- or do some writing
- or try some movement
- or rest
- or walk around the room a few times.

Ensure the client has time for emotions to resolve or feel settled. This may not happen immediately.

Review/Discussion:

- *Do you feel ready to talk about the experience?*
- *Is there anything you would like to share?*

Future Focus:

- *Are there any changes you need to make? Is there someone you want to help you?*
- *Are there any new plans or steps you would like to take?*
- *Should there be a plan for the future? For example, how will it be if or when you see them again?*

Discuss any new creative activities, engagement in hobbies or sports activities that could be alternatives to acting-out.

Ask if the client wants to share anything with parent(s), teachers or others, and ask if this needs support.

Activity 7.4 Emotion-Focused Process: *Finding My Animal Sounds*

Suggested Age Range: Approximately 7 to 12 years.

Materials: Drawing paper and crayons ready. Strong rhythmic background music may be helpful to support animal role-play (Steps 8 to 10).

Aim: Useful for clients who frequently exhibit traits of anger, but may not know specific, obvious causes; who may not be in touch with anger, but who exhibit acting-out behaviours.

Instruction:

Give an overview of the activity and its purpose.

Invite the client to: *Tune in to yourself, take a moment to be still. Take a few deep breaths.*

1. *Think of someone you are (or were) angry with or afraid of. I won't ask you to say who it is.*
2. *Can you create a large, quick SKETCH of their face? Make their eyes strong and use a dark crayon. It doesn't matter if you are good at drawing or not; just try a quick sketch to remind you of them.*
3. *Now, could you create a quick DRAWING of how you feel about this person? You can use lines, colours and shapes to show how you feel about them.*
4. Warm up – with bioenergetics:
   - shaking through the whole body – head to toes
   - the wood-chopper
   - *Get off my back!*
   - the *victory step* – saying *"Yes!"*.
5. *Place the drawing of the face on or against a wall, sitting opposite, or place it on a table to look down on. Focus on the face.*
6. *Mentally think what you would* really *like to say to this person. These might be things you would not say in real life – you can think anything.*
7. *Now could you whisper it? Speak the words so quietly that no one can hear. Can you focus on the face as you do this?*
   We will now try some magic breaths to change into some powerful animals: Take 3 big, full, slow magic breaths now.
8. *Imagine you are becoming a beautiful large dog, or perhaps a wolf? Feel your body change, get down on all fours if that helps you feel like the animal. Now in dog language say what you were whispering to the person out loud, as loud as you can.* (pause)
   Take 3 big magic breaths again. Make the breaths slow, full and then relax. These breaths are making you larger and stronger.

9. *Imagine you are becoming a tiger now – the largest, most powerful, most beautiful tiger in the world. Feel your claws, feel the strength in your back. Now say all those things you were thinking in tiger language, with tiger strength.*
   Take 3 more big magic breaths.
10. *Stand up. You are becoming an enormous majestic elephant – the largest in the world. Could you express yourself as an elephant? What sounds, what actions would you make? What would you say in elephant language?*
11. *STAND TALL and come back to being you now. Keep the animal energy inside you if you wish. Stretch, breathe, feel your energy and feelings now.*
    - *Turn away from the face.*
    - *Let your energy and strength be all through you.*
    - *Focus inside now, and feel that for a moment.*
12. *Turn to another page and quickly create another image of your feelings and energy now. Find the colours, lines, shapes that go with how you feel now after being the elephant.*
13. *Could you think about and write down anything you feel you need to actually say to this person (or needed to say in the past) – any information, boundaries, tell them what you want or don't want, what you will accept and what you will not accept.* (pause)
14. *How would you like to finish with the drawing of the face now? Do you want to talk about it? Leave it in the book? Add to it? Change it?*
15. With the client, reflect on drawings 2 (from Step 3) and 3 (from Step 12):
    - Are they similar or different?
    - Could the client find any words for the differences?
16. *Is there anything you would like to remember or write down about this activity?*

Discussion Options

- *How did you feel doing this activity?*
- *Was there a favourite step? Was there a difficult step?*
- *Is there anything you want to say about the person?*
- *Did you notice any changes in how you felt?*
- *Are there any steps you need to/want to take?*

Activity 7.5 Emotion-Focused Process: *The Dot on the Wall*

Suggested Age Range: From 7 to 14 years.

Materials: Small round stickers/dots, pen, cushions, tissues, optional energising background music.

Aim: This activity is designed to allow the young client to reverse the normal order of things. Usually, it is the bully/other person who holds the power. In this activity, the client imagines the other person as smaller than themselves. From the stronger position and in the confidential safe place of the counselling room, with qualified therapeutic support, the young person can have an experience of releasing restriction in emotional reactivity.

A key principle of this activity is the need to attend clearly to the integration phase. The aim is not to have the child stay in an elevated state of distress, but to allow the distress to be expelled and the client to return to a state of calmness.

Instructions

After discussion that helps identify the person – or group – they are reacting to and who the process will focus on, set up the work space for emotion processing: Large cushions, tissues, etc.

The client sits, facing the wall with pen, drawing book and crayons beside them. They close their eyes and tilt their head up, as if looking up at the person who is the focus of the process standing in front.

Process

1. Client is guided to take six full slow magic breaths. These breaths have special power. Each breath can shrink the person who is the focus of the process.
2. The client imagines the person becoming smaller with each breath,
   - they let their head move down at the same time (as if watching them shrinking)
   - the power of the person is being reduced
   - continue until the focus person is about the size of an ant.
3. Client puts out their hand and imagines the person, tiny now, on the palm of their hand. Facilitator places a dot about the size of a 10-cent coin on the client's hand. (Use adhesive round sticker.)
4. The client draws the face of the person on the dot.
5. Client sticks the dot low on the wall or floor in front of them so that they can look down on it.
6. With some empowering music in the background, the client creates an imaginary encounter and begins by telling the person:
   - all the things that they would like to say to the person, even if these are not things they would say in real life
   - then add as many adjectives and extra words as possible
   - repeat the expression
   - add all the other things they need or want to say – now or from the past.
7. Some deep breaths are encouraged.
8. The client is encouraged to express their feelings as fully as possible in the moment.

9. They are encouraged to repeat any key phrases, words or body movements. They could even make up a secret sign language.
10. If the client seems "stuck", invite them to talk about the stuck feeling and what might be behind it – e.g., loyalty issues, love, grief.
11. When they seem finished, they are invited to stand up, stretch and move (or dance).
12. Then the client is invited to tune-in to their body energy for a moment.
13. Ask them if they feel finished.
14. If they are feeling any positive feelings such as love or sadness, invite them to relax, feel their heart open and simply stay with this feeling.
15. When they are ready, the client removes the dot from the wall.
16. The client is asked how they would like to finish with the dot. (A variety of suggestions could be offered as possibilities, but avoid making "concrete" firm directions.)

Integration

The client is offered a range of integration activities to choose from, e.g.:

- go for a quick walk
- rest for a few minutes
- draw how they feel in a circle (mandala)
- make a picture with symbols or collage
- add a few words that go with how they felt after speaking to the dot.

Discuss any steps they need or want to take.

Discuss the challenges and support needed in taking these steps.

Discuss what will happen to the worksheet – it is usually kept in the counsellor's office.

Activity 7.6 Emotion-Focused Role-play: *Expressing Reactivity through Symbols*

Suggested Age Range: From 7 to 12 years.

Materials: Symbols, crayons, two sheets of A3-size drawing paper. Optional: Background music appropriate to the feelings being expressed for Step 6; followed by quiet, relaxing background music.

Aim: To discover, express and reduce reactive emotions, through role-play inspired by miniatures, using an imaginary encounter. This series of activities allows an enactment of emotion to vent, followed by reflection and integration. It is most useful, after establishing a good rapport with the client, after at least three or four sessions. It can contribute to reclaiming empowerment.

Note: These types of emotion-focused activities are suitable for relatively stable clients.

Provide an overview and rationale for the activity.

Focus

1. Clarify any reactive feelings the client feels they need to, or want to, deal with.
2. The client externalises the person or situation they have strong reactive feelings about through drawing a quick picture of the person or situation.

They are invited to share how they feel while creating the picture.

3. The client is asked to select three symbols that, to them, represent the reactive feelings they need to deal with – for example, Anger, sadness, jealousy, happiness, a feeling of fear, danger, etc.

E.g.: *Could you choose the three angriest symbols?*

4. Discuss symbol choice:

   - *Can you say what you liked or didn't like about the symbols?*
   - *Can you tell me anything about them and their feelings?*
   - *Can you imagine anything about their lives?*
   - *Which is the angriest? Which is next in anger, and which is the least angry?*

Process

5. Bioenergetic games as warm-up:

Client and counsellor stand up and play with these activities together.

- Shaking the whole body from head to toe. Is there an image that helps the shaking?
- "Bound and free" – alternating tension and breaking free – Squeeze body tight, hold breath, burst free.
- Grounding in legs – bend knees, put the weight of your whole body on one leg for about a minute, then shake the leg, then move your weight onto the other leg.

6. Invite the client to stand in front of the drawing of the person or situation they react to.

Role-play, moving and sounding or speaking, as each of the three selected symbols, in order of intensity, starting with the least intense.

- *What posture would you take to help you feel like the symbols?*
- *What would you do with your hands? Your feet?*
- *What expression would you have on your face?*
- *Could you exaggerate all that?*

- *Could you look at the eyes of the face while you pretend to be this symbol?*
- *You can move and make sounds, and direct them towards the drawing.*

Counsellor gives positive feedback and encouragement during the role-play.

During the role-play, the client is invited to find any sounds, try out words, and actions towards the drawing.

Encourage the client to expand the movements, sounds and any words to assist the expressive release.

Emotionally appropriate background music might help give permission for entering the drama.

Integration

7. After role-play, suggest the client:

- *Stand up, turn away from the drawing of the person or situation now.*
- *Tune-in to yourself. What do you notice inside right now?*
- *Is there a feeling or a mood now?* (pause)

8. *Can you select another two or three symbols for the feeling, mood or energy inside now?*

- *On a fresh page, could you arrange the new symbols into a picture or story?*
- *Which would be close? Which would be further apart? Which way would they be facing?*
- *Could you add colours and lines that help show how they feel, and how they might connect?*
- *See if you would like to add any words or comments?*

9. *Would you like to share what you have just created? Is there anything you would like to say about this arrangement, about this picture, and what happened before it?*
10. *Is there some way you would like to finish off with the first drawing – of the person or group or situation?*
11. Consider if a further integration activity would be useful, e.g., discussion, drawing, mandala creation, shaping something in play dough or clay, or writing a summary of experiences, or simply resting. The client may like to take a photograph of their creation.

Strategies

12. Help the client formulate any new strategies or recognise any supports that may be needed in relation to the focus person(s) or situation, and for managing any future frustration or stress.

References

Armstrong, T. (1994). *Multiple intelligences in the classroom*. Association for Supervision and Curriculum Development.

Bowlby, J. (1988). Developmental psychiatry comes of age. *The American Journal of Psychiatry*, *145*(1), 1–10.

Cicchetti, D., Ackerman, B. P., & Izard, C. E. (1995). Emotions and emotion regulation in developmental psychopathology. *Development and Psychopathology*, *7*, 1–10. https://doi.org/10.1017/S0954579400006301

Dhabhar, F. S. (2013). Psychological stress and immunoprotection versus immunopathology in the skin. *Clinics in Dermatology*, *31*(1), 18–30.

Fosha, D. (2000). *The transforming power of affect: A model for accelerated change*. Basic Books.

Freud, S. (1915). Instincts and their vicissitudes. *Standard Edition*, *14*(1957), 109–140.

Gardner, H. (2006). *Multiple intelligences. New horizons*. Basic Books.

Greene, J. W., & Walker, L. S. (1997). Psychosomatic problems and stress in adolescence. *Pediatric Clinics of North America*, *44*(6), 1557–1572.

Greenberg, L. S. (2002). Integrating an emotion-focused approach to treatment into psychotherapy integration. *Journal of Psychotherapy Integration*, *12*(2), 154–189. https://doi.org/10.1037/1053-0479.12.2.154

Greenberg, L. S. (2004). Emotion–focused therapy. *Clinical Psychology & Psychotherapy: An International Journal of Theory & Practice*, *11*(1), 3–16.

Greenberg, L. S. (2006). Emotion-focused therapy: A synopsis. *Journal of Contemporary Psychotherapy*, *36*, 87–93.

Greenberg, L. S. (2015). *Emotion-focused therapy: Coaching clients to work through their feelings* (2nd ed.). American Psychological Association. https://doi.org/10.1037/14692-000

Holian, L. (2001). *Metacognition: Highlighting the importance of emotional reflection and expression* (Unpublished master's project). Monash University.

Kadzikowska-Wrzosek, R. (2012). Perceived stress, emotional ill-being and psychosomatic symptoms in high school students: The moderating effect of self-regulation competences. *Archives of Psychiatry and Psychotherapy*, *3*, 25–33.

Kalff, D.M. (2003). *Sandplay - A psychotherapeutic approach to the psyche*. Temenos Press.

Kelly, C., Molcho, M., Doyle, P., & Gabhainn, S. N. (2010). Psychosomatic symptoms among schoolchildren. *International Journal of Adolescent Medicine and Health*, *22*(2), 229–236.

Lowenfeld, M. (1935). *Play in childhood*. Gollancz.

McEwen, B. S. (2007). Physiology and neurobiology of stress and adaptation: Central role of the brain. *Physiological Reviews*, *87*(3), 873–904.

O'Brien, P., & Burnett, P. (2000). Counselling children using a multiple intelligence framework. *British Journal of Guidance and Counselling*, *28*(3), 353–371. https://doi.org/10.1080/03069880050118993

Payne, W. L. (1985). *A study of emotion: Developing emotional intelligence; self-integration; relating to fear, pain and desire* (Dissertation). The Union for Experimenting Colleges and Universities.

Pearson, M. (2003). Guidance officer and counsellor perspectives on using expressive therapies to support students. *Australian Journal of Guidance & Counselling, 13*(2), 205–224.

Pearson, M. (2006). *The inner space program: A proactive groupwork program for emotional literacy and student well-being.* Expressive Therapies Australia.

Pearson, M., & Wilson, H. (2001). *Sandplay and symbol work: Emotional healing and personal development with children, adolescents and adults.* ACER Press.

Pearson, M., & Wilson, H. (2008). Using expressive counselling tools to enhance emotional literacy, emotional wellbeing and resilience: Improving therapeutic outcomes with Expressive Therapies. *Counselling, Psychotherapy and Health, 4*(1), 1–19.

Pearson, M., & Wilson, H. (2012). Soothing spaces and healing places: Is there an ideal counselling room design? *Psychotherapy in Australia, 18*(3), 46–53.

Sharp, P. (2001). *Nurturing emotional literacy: A practical guide for teachers, parents and those in the caring professions.* David Fulton Publishers.

Simmons, S. (2006). Living the questions: Existential intelligence in the context of holistic art education. *Visual Arts Research, 32*(1), 41–52.

Spendlove, D. (2008). *Emotional literacy.* Continuum

Stien, P., & Kendall, J. C. (2014). *Psychological trauma and the developing brain: Neurologically based interventions for troubled children.* Routledge.

Tereba, H. (1999). *Time travellers* (Unpublished masters thesis). Queensland University of Technology.

8 Trauma-Informed Expressive Therapies

In this chapter, the aim is to share some of what ET can offer in support of clients who carry a legacy from trauma. This chapter contains activities specifically developed for young clients in recovery from trauma. We are not aiming to introduce the wide and varied field of trauma treatment. The last 20 years have seen rapid growth in understanding the needs of traumatised young clients. In addition, a significant body of evidence highlights the contribution creative arts therapies make to positive therapeutic outcomes (e.g., Carey, 2006; Malchiodi, 2020; Perry, 2006; van Westrhenen et al., 2017).

A significant number of ET activities (with some very clear exceptions – see page 179) can be useful in the work of trauma recovery once a sense of safety and rapport has been established. The invitational, person-centred way of working with ET makes it suitable for a very wide range of client presentations. In essence, activities that do not deliberately provoke experiences, but allow a spontaneous "playing out" of stresses, are ideal. There are many ET activities that specifically support grounding and stabilisation. All appropriate activities work best when offered in an invitational way – an attitude and processes that provide an atmosphere of autonomy and choice for clients.

Recognising Trauma

What is already known is traumatic events have the potential to overwhelm human adaptation. In general, a trauma involves threats to life or bodily integrity, or a close encounter with violence and death (Herman, 2015). The outcomes include severe disturbances in cognitive and emotional processing. Deficits in information-processing ultimately disrupt integrated neural processing. In other words, clarity of thought, behaviour and emotional expression may all be out of balance. Therapy for a client who has experienced trauma, especially younger clients, starts with creating an atmosphere of safety. This happens most easily and effectively in a context of predictable, respectful relationships. The recovery journey begins, ideally, when therapeutic work offers a client psychological safety, a capacity to play and a sense of choice (Perry, 2006). Recommendations from multi-modal approaches in trauma

DOI: 10.4324/9781003671879-8

treatment indicate growing interest in applying ET methods (e.g., Garrett, 2020; Jaaniste & Perry, 2021).

For a child, trauma disconnects them from relational resources and restricts their capacity to pay attention. Trauma negatively affects social skills development and can disrupt peer relationships (Barton, Gonzalez, Tomlinson, 2012). We could say they feel "cut adrift" at a time they need connection, but find it difficult to utilise reasoning and logic to modify reactions or behaviour. Heightened arousal states mean there is a lower likelihood of learning from consequences.

In light of traumatic experiences, a child may become highly anxious and unable to switch off from feelings of anxiety. The result is deprivation from experiences essential for normal growth, i.e., play, relaxation and enjoyment of nurturance (Barton, Gonzalez, Tomlinson, 2012). Creating opportunities for these three experiences is central in ET practice. Expressive therapists employ playful interventions that promote spontaneity, use and teach multiple ways of achieving relaxation, and aim to use the therapeutic relationship to provide authentic experiences of care and nurturance.

There are a range of conditions that call for trauma-informed support. Some clients are influenced by significant stress and shock. Others experience stress so overwhelming it is classified as traumatic. Post-traumatic stress emerges when stress resulting from trauma remains ongoing (at least for a month) (Pynoos et al., 2009). The term "Post-traumatic stress disorder" (PTSD) is used when ongoing stress impacts or interrupts functioning and daily life.

Less acknowledged in the therapeutic literature is "Prolonged duress stress disorder" (Scott & Stradling, 1994); harder to identify, yet quite common. PDSD can arise when a person has experienced pressure by or from others in a negative way over time, so that this seemingly permanent stress impacts daily life and behaviour. These clients may seem to have no immediately obvious cause for stress responses, but display a number of PTSD-like symptoms. Some of the causes of prolonged stress during the developmental years include, among others, neglect, chronic illness and a dysfunctional family system. For PDSD, therapeutic processes will often focus on the development of resilience (Marsh, 2003).

During Traumatic Events

Trauma-sensitive therapists aim to be alert to in-session clues from the client that reconnection with previously dissociated traumatic experiences may be underway. This means a natural struggle between dissociation and reconnection may be active. Somatic indicators and physiological changes in the client, such as attentional changes, postural and gestural changes and changes in facial expression, may become active as trauma experiences re-emerge into awareness in the here-and-now. Our observations may guide us to invite a client to note their internal experience and communicate it, if they are willing to continue. Young clients can exhibit diversionary tactics; for example, distancing, claiming boredom, changing topics and changing or focusing on their choice of media. It is ideal to go with this "flow". As part of ET, we subscribe to Rothchild's (2010) concept of "putting on the brakes", supporting the client's need to slow down their process, gently extending their tolerance for exposure. Reconnection with uncomfortable sensations, feelings and memories is not "coached" nor provoked, but allowed to emerge once there is a reliable sense of Herman's (2015) first phase of stabilisation.

During trauma, respiration and heart rate increase; blood is sent away from the skin into muscles to enable rapid movement (Rothschild, 2010). We may observe a pale face and deeper or faster breathing. Automatic survival mechanisms, instantaneous reflexes, are activated during trauma and may account for somatic and psychological changes within a therapy session. Speech can be suppressed during trauma. During a traumatic episode, the hippocampus becomes partially suppressed, and cognitive processing is inhibited. The result may be that in session, a client may communicate in a tangential way. Mobilisation of the body for fight, flight or freeze during trauma means similar responses can occur in the therapy room. In therapy, verbal communication may become limited or completely stalled when traumatic experiences are discussed or activated. Dissociation from fear and pain during trauma may become a somewhat permanent state, making internal awareness less possible or agreeable. Therefore, our usual invitation to "tune in and see what is happening inside" may feel inappropriate, fear-inducing, or even threatening to that part of the client seeking to self-protect.

Additionally, trauma induces guilt and shame that may "flood" a person at some later stage. Difficulty in self-forgiveness may be evident, along with fear of judgemental counsellor responses, experienced as shame. What this means is that it can take a long time for a person to feel safe enough to self-disclose. Shame has been identified as a factor in the development and maintenance of PTSD (Au et al, 2016) and therapeutic approaches that promote self-compassion have shown some promise for reducing the shame burden (Au et al, 2016).

Two Types of Memory

Humans have both explicit memory and implicit memory, and Expressive Therapies can support work with both. Explicit (declarative) memory relates to facts, concepts and ideas (Rothschild, 2010). It enables the telling of one's life story, narrating events, putting experience into words and extracting meaning. Implicit (procedural) memory involves procedures and internal states that are automatic and may bypass language. Procedural memory operates unconsciously unless made conscious through creating a bridge to explicit memory in order to make sense of what is remembered. Healing and neural integration involve developing links between both implicit and explicit memory (Malchiodi, 2020).

Traumatic memories are said to be stored implicitly in the brain's right hemisphere, making verbal expression of trauma memories more difficult (Schiffer, Teicher, & Papanicolaou, 1995). In reducing the lived emotional and psychological legacy of trauma, integration of distressing events is enhanced through engaging in activities that support bridging between explicit and implicit memory. For example, expressive writing and journaling; symbol work; creation of narratives, and timeline activities.

With its focus on developing emotional and somatic awareness, ET activities offer an ideal pathway for recovery. Expression that is not specifically dependent on language is most likely to be effective. The use of therapeutic activities that are primarily non-verbal is recommended to allow contact with, and expression of, implicit memories (Steele & Malchiodi, 2012). A logical response, then, is that a range of non-verbal therapeutic activities is highly likely to support positive therapeutic progress for trauma-informed care.

The brain processes perceptions and stores them as separate thoughts, emotions, images, sensations and behavioural impulses (Rothschild, 2010). Each impulse could, therefore, be considered a "doorway" for clients – a starting point for therapy. The greater the significance and higher the emotional charge (both positive and negative), the more likely a piece of information will be stored. One of the keys to effective therapy is, therefore, skilfully and gently accessing the emotional charge. Being able to process emotions is one way to reduce some of the "charge". ET activities, with their multiple ways to help bring the client back into the present, and find "voice" to express and ultimately reduce emotional stress.

Clients recovering from trauma need support that provides opportunities for them to become "alive" in the current moment and rebuild agency and control in their lives. The "need" for control becomes paramount (Steele & Malchiodi, 2012), so inviting client reflection on preferences, having their choices respected, gives opportunities to rehearse and strengthen rebuilding agency. Working with an attitude of invitation means ET activities are highly effective in rehearsing what choice feels like.

Using ET with Traumatised Clients

The importance of developing rapport and trust has already been emphasised in trauma care. "The more secure children feel, the more time, energy and inclination they have to seek and make sense. Whereas fear constricts, safety expands the range of exploration" (Cameron & Maginn, 2009, p. 28). Our therapeutic attitude, capacity for attunement and ability to offer and create a safe psychological space become paramount. Children and young people who have experienced trauma need a therapeutic environment where they can safely attend to vulnerabilities and heal – a place and space that meets their emotional need to feel safe (Barton et al., 2012).

Expressive arts activities have been shown to effectively treat trauma (e.g., Sosin et al, 2022). Through skilled understanding and multiple tools for reflection and expression, implicit aspects of trauma memories – that are otherwise challenging to tolerate – can gradually be put into words. Additionally, the mindfulness activities incorporated into ET can add to increased cognitive flexibility and emotional and physiological regulation in response to trauma activation (Strand & Stige, 2021). As ET promotes a client's expression, their somatic and emotional awareness, within a stable, caring and invitational therapeutic relationship, means ET becomes ideal for work within a trauma-informed therapeutic programme.

Trauma-sensitive care recommendations while using ET frameworks and activities include:

1. Set up the counselling room to support a feeling of safety, with privacy, accessibility, beauty, some order – as well as just a little chaos (the combination can imply a sense of freedom for the client).
2. To begin, we develop rapport with the client and engender trust in the therapist and their consulting space. In some cases, this may include reviewing previous therapeutic encounters considered unsuccessful or that contributed to anxiety or a lower level of trust.
3. If necessary, help reduce "performance anxiety" in the counselling encounter. Emphasise that the client can't be wrong. Having choice in relation to discussion topics, activities, levels and depth of self-expression and self-revelation may build a sense of self-confidence, and the notion that choice is possible about what is discussed.
4. Allow clients to experience consistency within counselling sessions. Plan to follow the same, or very similar, steps and similar activities within the first few sessions. This supports feeling safe – there are no surprises.
5. Offer some grounding activities that invite somatic re-connection while simultaneously understanding that clients who have developed protective disassociation may resist invitations to bring awareness to the body. For example, for grounding, invite a client to see if they can feel: Their feet on the floor, their breath flowing in and out, etc.
6. As the alliance strengthens, discern appropriateness and timing to offer emotion-focused activities. For example, after establishing relational safety, provide opportunities to safely externalise and defuse reactivity.
7. An invitation to use miniatures and metaphors supports safe articulation of difficult experiences. This process allows clients to externalise, symbolise, and keep experiences at a manageable and tolerable emotional distance. Allow oscillation between positive reinforcement and approaching vulnerabilities.
8. Develop within the client a connection to a safe retreat place, and normalise the concept of going at their pace through "putting the brakes on" (Rothschild, 2010) (e.g., see activity page 217).
9. In the initial stages of the work, provide some stimulation of communication through techniques that do not depend on cognition or language

sophistication. Conversation catalysts may include sentence starters, selection and arrangement of miniatures in response to either spontaneous attraction or in response to questions posed, graphic expression, music selection and silent games.

10. Offer multiple ways to externalise beliefs, thoughts, memories, feelings or body sensations through drawing, miniature selection and arrangement.
11. Focus on identifying strengths and indicators of resilience in early and late stages of therapy (e.g., see pages 201 and 204). Focus on ways to assist the client to identify, articulate and be reminded of strengths.
12. Once a strong alliance has been established, find ways to gradually link and integrate implicit and explicit memory. For example, engage a client in reflection about any meaning that arises from spontaneously chosen miniatures. Select activities that support connection between right and left hemisphere functioning for effective integration: For example, follow up emotion-focused activities with reflective review (e.g., summarising highlights of the session).
13. Once contact with affect has happened, follow up with integration when the client is invited to say what meaning they make of the experience. Plan to allow sufficient time for integration and closure. (Stages 4 and 5 – see page 45).
14. Endeavour to work holistically, inviting the client to move between somatic awareness, emotional awareness and cognitive awareness. Also make time and emotional space if a client raises any spiritual concerns. Allow times of distraction, diversion and wait for an appropriate moment to return their attention to the topic at hand. This process follows some of the principles of the Dual Process Model of coping with bereavement (Schut, 1999).
15. Develop your trust in the client's pacing for emotional processing and their readiness to move on from stabilisation to reconnect with their experience (Session stage 2). An attitude of patience within ourselves is imperative to support further resolution of distress.
16. Bring a focus on resilience development (page 201), and provide positive feedback when the client demonstrates self-management or uses the Inner-Life Skills (page 180).
17. Furthermore, develop in yourself an optimistic future focus. Our optimism can influence a client's optimism. Initiation of a client's hope can contribute to positive therapeutic outcomes (Bartholomew, Joy & Gundel, 2021).

Developing Resilience

Resilience has been described as "the individual's capacity for adapting successfully and continuing to function competently under stress and adversity" (Howe, 2005, p. 219). Howe also claims that "experiences of sensitive, mind-engaging and secure attachments promote resilience" (2005, p. 219). In everyday terms, resilience usually means "bouncing back" from difficult experiences. Basic resilience is developed through caring and positive relationships (American Psychological Association website). This suggests that counsellors are well placed to support young clients to develop resilience.

Concluding a study of resilience, Masten (2001), summarised "the great threats to human development" (p. 234). She identified threats that adversely influence adaptive processes such as brain development and cognition, caregiver and child relationships, regulation of emotion and behaviour and the motivation for learning and interacting with the environment. Masten's analysis of resilience studies leads to the identification of a reasonably tight set of factors associated with resilience. These include connections with competent and caring adults, cognitive and self-regulation skills, positive views of self and motivation to be effective in the environment. There are significant personality factors that distinguish a resilient child from those who become overwhelmed by negative factors (Rak & Patterson, 1996). These include an "active approach toward problem-solving, an ability to gain others' positive attention, an optimistic view of their experiences, an ability to maintain a positive vision of a meaningful life, the ability to be alert and autonomous, a tendency to seek novel experiences, in addition to a proactive perspective" (p. 369).

The road to resilience is likely to lead a young person through facing emotional distress and involves acquiring revised behaviours and perspectives that can be learned and developed (APA, n.d.). Having an aim of helping clients gently overcome a natural or cultural tendency towards experiential avoidance may prove valuable. Developing resilience is a personal journey, and an approach to building resilience that works for one person might not work for another. Extra-therapeutic use of a wide range of "cultural resources" is recommended (McLeod, 2018). These resources are activities that support a person's wellbeing and may include hobbies, literature, group experiences and self-care practices. Counsellors have a role in guiding clients of all ages towards greater resilience and supporting them to recognise which cultural resources might be most beneficial for support beyond their time in the therapy room.

As there is no single form for an effective resilience-promoting intervention, an integrative way of providing counselling support is preferable. The strongest resilience-building interventions develop psychosocial skills and support key relationships (Graber, Pichon, & Carabine, 2015). Therefore, increasing clients' capacities with both the intrapersonal and interpersonal intelligences (Gardner, 2006) is recommended (see more on page 12), within a person-focused therapeutic framework (Mearns & Thorne, 2000). Furthermore, a therapeutic goal (when positive family relationships have been identified) of encouraging clients to strengthen ties with family and friends is positively indicated (Graber et al, 2015). Resilience interventions may also have effects on physiological functioning (e.g., Feder et al., 2009; Gallo et al., 2009; Wu et al., 2013). Key features of effective resilience interventions include the use of strengths, emotional support and meaning-making (Graber et al, 2015). A range of appropriate options for therapeutic response includes strengths-based approaches (Duncan, 2010), the incorporation of self-discovery activities (Pearson & Wilson, 2009) and integration of existential reflection (Cooper, 2016).

Meaning in life has also been identified as a predictor of resilience and well-being (Lightsey, 2006). Increase in life meaning predicted a positive change in mental health (Jacobson, 2002). Meaning emerges through a sense of belonging, doing and understanding (King, 2004). Counsellors have clear roles that involve generating experiences for young clients of belonging, engaging and being active in sessions, with hoped-for moments of self-understanding (Lightsey, 2006). ET approaches include "doing" elements that enable young clients to engage, reflect and integrate and make sense of their experiences. An expressive therapist aims to remain focused, attuned and caring, in some ways reflecting an ideal, early, parent-child connection (Pearson & Wilson, 2009). This carries echoes of Rogers' (1951) emphasis on creating, in therapy, a relationship characterised by unconditional positive regard as an integral ingredient to support effective psychological change.

Positive emotions, such as gratitude, interest, love, support coping. Positive emotions not only put the mind at ease but have the capacity to create relaxation in the body, even lowering heart rate and blood pressure (Fredrickson et al., 2003). Findings from research suggest that positive emotions experienced after a crisis can provide a buffer against depression (Fredrickson et al., 2003), and may naturally emerge during the therapeutic process. Recurring experiences of positive emotions contribute to building resilience. Positive emotions such as joy, interest, pride and love are able to expand the range of options for behaviour (Greenberg, 2002), which in turn builds longer-lasting internal resources.

The authors have frequently observed that when clients can be supported to process difficult or "negative" emotions, their overall emotional state transforms to a much more positive and regulated state. ET encourages this "working through" of emotions in a safe way, allowing metaphor, symbolism and projection to create safety and some distance from overwhelming emotions. Imagery as a way to support growth in resilience brings a tendency to generate positive emotions that foster self-soothing. The development of emotional literacy and skills for managing emotions developed through experiences with ET activities strengthens this ability to be able to draw on and experience positive experiences.

Abuse, ET and Children

A key factor in helping children who have experienced abuse is the presence of someone who can offer unconditional, positive regard (Doyle, 2003), a therapeutic relational stance first advocated by Rogers (1980). Doyle (2003) found that children who believe they can have some control and attribute any success and achievement to their own abilities are likely to do better than children who believe they have no control.

For maltreated children, having or creating healthy self-affirming friendships can lead to increased self-esteem, less loneliness, and feelings of greater acceptance than in those without friends (Bolger & Patterson, 2003). The indication is that ET group work activities can support the development of new bonds, in addition to support for social skill development. In some cases, moving from individual sessions to participation in ET groups for personal development may add to recovery and resilience-building.

ET has been created specifically to foster and confirm experiences of achievement, albeit in small, regular doses. Clients experience achievement (during activities) and directorship (through choice) in sessions. The client is invited to participate, construct, create, play, manipulate and control media and observe their creations. The final results provide tangible evidence of resourcefulness; something emerged from within them.

Having new images of self (being able to mentalise self) supports positive therapeutic outcomes for a client (Siegel, 2007). Howe (2005) suggests that a secure child's growing ability to "mentalise" and make sense of themselves and others provides access to high levels of resilience. Making sense of self and others, access to intrapersonal intelligence, having a revised or new image of self: All emerge with relative ease when ET is the prime facilitator of recovery.

Mindfulness and Resilience

Mindfulness has a variety of definitions, including "paying attention in a particular way: on purpose, in the present moment, and nonjudgmentally" (Kabat-Zinn, 1994, p. 4), and "awareness of present experience with acceptance" (Germer, 2005, p. 7). Over the last twenty years mindfulness has been incorporated within psychodynamic and cognitive-behavioural approaches (Mace, 2007), as well as creative arts and expressive therapies. Mindfulness emphasises the importance of experience over knowledge. The practice focuses on generating non-judgemental awareness in the here and now, and has significant implications for integration in therapy. Hinterkopf (1998) recommended a Focusing activity to support clients' reconnection with spirituality; a simple process to activate an individual existential search. The aim was to generate new experiences of meaning and personal satisfaction, which have both been shown to contribute to resilience (Lightsey, 2006).

Perceiving emotional, somatic and cognitive experiences more closely and clearly means a client can be supported to extend tolerance and become less habitual and automatic in reactive tendencies. We have found combining an attitude of mindfulness with creative arts approaches – in particular expressing internal experiences through colour, lines, shapes and images – enhances the overall effectiveness of therapy. Focusing attention internally provides building blocks for new neural pathways (Siegel, 2007), an overall aim of psychotherapy.

Somatic and emotional focusing are used throughout ET and aim to generate a pathway that enhances client self-awareness for more effective processing of issues. We have found that mindfulness activities for young clients, as compared to adult activities, generally require shortened timeframes and are more likely to succeed when they include some movement and artistic expression. This has also been observed by Coholic et al., (2009). Clay et al (2024) found that a brief mindfulness activity enhanced creativity in the production of photographs that were more creative, complex, abstract, expressive and higher in emotional valence than a control group. A 12-hour mindfulness and mask-making programme supported young people to reduce their stress and anxiety (Lindsey, Robertson & Lindsey, 2018). Research over the last twenty years also indicates positive outcomes from adapting mindfulness meditations for young people (e.g., Perry-Parrish et al., 2016; Rempel, 2012). In Stage Two of the ET 5-Stage Model for session planning (see page 36), a self-awareness focus begins to develop a client's confidence with tolerating mindfulness.

Promoting mindfulness practice for therapists in training has an influence on the treatment results of their clients (Grepmair et al., 2007). Trainee therapists who participated in a mindfulness meditation course had significantly higher evaluations for individual therapy on scales related to clarification and problem-solving perspectives (Grepmair et al., 2007). Clients of the group that practised meditation showed greater symptom reduction than the therapists in training who did not practise meditation. An obvious implication is that we practise what we preach, or teach. ET activities that enhance ability with mindfulness can be found in Chapter 9.

There are, of course, cautions in relation to offering mindfulness to clients. Binda, Greco and Morone (2022) point out that adverse outcomes from mindfulness most often relate to extended meditation practices. In ET, playful and time-limited mindfulness activities are offered. The adult literature has reported that mindfulness meditation could potentially re-traumatise people who have a history of post-traumatic stress through creating too strong a window of awareness before establishing a secure enough base (Binda, Greco, & Morone, 2022). Our recommendation is that the ET invitational approach prevails when beginning to offer a mindfulness focus activity. Monitor the client's responses as you proceed. Let the client know they can call "stop" at any time. Provide ample opportunity for a client to discuss any unsettling observations, provide an activity that supports some processing of discomfort (e.g., see page 136 and 162).

Relationship in Therapeutic Outcomes

A factor common to all effective therapies is relationship, including "warmth and attention, understanding, and encouragement" (Lambert, 2005, p. 151). These aspects of relating are seen as central to the effectiveness of therapy and play an active role in client improvement. (Lambert, 2005; Seewald, & Rief, 2024). Some of the therapeutic elements – common to a wide range of therapies – include "identification with the therapist, mitigation of isolation, positive relationship, reassurance, release of tension, therapeutic alliance, therapist and client's active participation, therapist warmth (and respect, empathy, acceptance, genuineness), trust" (Lambert, 2005, p. 173). These elements remind us again that how we are may be just as crucial to outcomes as what we do or say or invite a client to engage with. We are also reminded by Terr (1994) that clients who have experienced trauma and have low levels of resilience may depend on the therapeutic relationship as their foundation for developing resilience and safety in the world. Therapeutic success for these clients may be the establishment of the supportive relationship with the therapist, with limited focus on further processing of trauma.

Within counselling, the teaching and modelling of behaviours that support a client to self-manage problems and stress is recommended by Rak and Patterson (1996). A facilitator stance of nurturance that conveys unconditional positive regard is again recommended. These researchers suggest the use of groups to develop resiliency skills, along with the use of role-play and creative imagery that support improved self-expression. Within ET, self-expression is seen as a central focus, a key to mental health.

We recommend that counsellors relate to young clients with an underlying aim to support re-discovering and reclaiming resourcefulness. Resilience can be enhanced when a client gains a sense of satisfaction with their level of involvement in the therapeutic process. The positive assumptions that underlie a therapeutic relationship encourage a client's ability to work through issues and build resilience. If a therapist relates to a client with a certainty that the person has the resources to work through their issues, and if they relate to clients with optimism and the assumption they can contribute and gain clarity, the client may also feel optimistic that they can do it; they have an experience of feeling successful.

Components of Resilience Development

Dignity: Counsellors aim to promote the dignity of the client. This means offering unconditional emotional support, validating feelings and experience, while obviously not approving destructive behaviours. To say "the client is the client", means being aware of their goals, their rights and their wishes, and noting if these diverge or are at odds with parent or carer goals. Part of upholding the client's dignity is offering freedom through presenting choice: Choice of topic focus and choice of therapeutic activity. Offering choice enhances engagement, conveys respect and can enhance creativity (Baloche, 1996).

Client Preferences: Adapting to client preferences and natural strengths leads us to provide multiple ways for the client to tell their story and process challenges. That adaptation can be supported by assessing clients from a multiple intelligences perspective (Pearson, 2011), identifying their natural strengths and initially offering activities that correspond to their preferred or natural intelligences. See more on this on page 8.

Trauma-informed practice prioritises the need for us to co-operate with and support a client's need to feel safe and secure (Chafouleas et al., 2016).

Respecting a need for self-protection means we allow time to discover and understand the logical causes of any resistance, apprehension or defences. We work with an attitude of respect for a client's timing for the development of trust and willingness to participate in counselling.

Hope: Hope is an important contributor to therapeutic effectiveness (Asay & Lambert, 1999; Hubble & Miller, 2004; Lambert, 1992), and plays an integral role in client wellbeing (Menninger, 1959; Monk et al., 1997; Yalom, 2001). Hope orientates towards the future and provides motivation to envision new possibilities and create pathways around obstacles (O'Hara, 2025). Snyder, Michael and Cheavens (1999) suggest that hope serves as a unifying framework in therapy and that well-documented positive placebo effects are essentially the result of hope. ET practice works from an optimistic stance. Counsellor hope and expectation of client growth and development will inform how we work and can be transmitted to a client. With hope that counselling can help a significant factor in positive outcomes, an expressive therapist aims to help grow client optimism about attending counselling. One way to support this is to begin the quest for identifying client goals. Another is to allow implicit hope to emerge through creative activities that can reflect back to the client some hopeful aspects of self and some new ways forward.

Understanding Acting-Out: Our understanding and responding to acting-out as an indication of the inherent drive towards exorcising stress, reclaiming resilience and achieving emotional balance – even though it does not achieve this – will support a non-judgemental attitude. It seems natural for the mind, body and emotion system to attempt resolution of what has been absorbed, or has not been resolved. Following this, we can use the client's style of acting-out, or withdrawing, as a guide to plan therapeutic activities. For example, if their acting-out has been quite physical, using bioenergetic games may contribute to resolution. If their style is more a type of withdrawal, offering quiet, self-reflection writing prompts may help (see page 108 to 110).

Acceptance: Sometimes offering unconditional positive regard may mean we have to accept client interpretations of events – accepting their narrative, even if it does not match the facts as we know them. Aiming to establish the veracity of all client statements is less important than establishing a collaborative working alliance. Many young clients initially interpret the need for counselling as a sign of blame or judgement. Experiencing acceptance from us may be a first step in diminishing their self-criticism.

Non-Interpretive Stance: Help clients discover their own meaning in their artwork, projective images and arrangements of miniatures. Avoid imposing interpretations. Can we use our attempts at interpretation to formulate questions for the client that simulate their self-reflection and self-discovery? What we want to avoid is reinforcing a client's assumption that others know best, are experts about them. Being provided with scaffolding to reflect and finding their own meanings contributes to building resilience.

Strategies and Activities to Support Resilience

The building of resilience is regarded as essential to reduce mental health problems in young people (Oliver et al., 2006). Links between resilience research and neuroscience have been established in the context of interventions that improve executive functions: Inhibitory control, planning skills, problem-solving skills, emotional regulation and attentional capacities (Greenberg, 2006). Stage 5 of our ET session planning model includes a focus on planning and problem solving (see page 46).

To summarise, ET supports the development of a young client's resilience through an invitational, warm, accepting relationship. To encourage this relationship, we provide self-esteem-building activities, offer self-discovery opportunities, aim to nurture a client's positive view of self, support their formulation of problem-solving methods, and offer both some challenge and a high degree of support for emotional expression. ET methods provide multiple ways for clients to hold trauma at a workable distance, and yet begin to work through distress in symbolic and metaphorical ways. For clients who are ready and able, ET allows them to approach and work through difficult emotions, make sense of what happened and consolidate a focus on moving forward in life.

PRACTICAL ACTIVITIES FOR TRAUMA WORK

Activity 8.1 Visualisation for Grounding and Stabilisation: *The Peaceful Park*

This peaceful story could help you feel calm. It might be useful if going to sleep at night is not easy. See if you can imagine yourself in the story.

I have some words, a story, to help your imagination. See if you would be able to let the pictures emerge in your mind.

Pictures that go with the story might come from your imagination and show themselves. I hope that listening to the story and imagining the pictures will help you relax and feel restful. If you feel this activity is not helpful, please do let me know straight away.

Would you like to rest in a comfy chair? Sometimes closing your eyes or softening your eyelids helps you listen to the story and imagine pictures more clearly. You might like to try that out?

So, let's start? Imagine you are in a beautiful park you know well. It is a fine warm afternoon. It is a large park, with plenty of space for everyone. Your friends and family are playing nearby, but you have taken a moment to relax lie on some grass and be quiet.

See if you are resting on your back, or on your side. The grass is warm and soft. You can see blue sky, and you can hear your friends nearby.

There are tall trees and green bushes around you, and lots of bright flowers. Birds are flying about and singing in the trees. See if you can imagine their songs.

You have been watching the trees moving in the breeze, swaying from side to side. You see the branches bend and dance, as the leaves flutter, way up above you. Sometimes you wish you could be riding up there on those branches, free like a bird, swaying on the breeze.

Behind the trees you see blue sky and white clouds. And now you watch the clouds drift by. As they float across the sky they change shape. See if you can imagine the clouds floating by. What shapes are they making?

Now you listen to the birds. They are singing to each other, and it seems like they are also singing just for you. What do you think the birds would say if they could sing to you in human language?

You are resting warm and comfortable on the grass. And soon it will be time to go back to your friends.

You close your eyes for a moment. You can feel the warm air on your skin, you take a few deep breaths. You rest here for a while, enjoying the warmth.

When you feel ready, you might like to bring your focus back into this room and have a stretch. Open your eyes, and look around.

On the art paper, would you be able to create an image from the story that can help you show the feeling of being in the park? Or maybe you could explore just using colours and shapes to show how it felt?

Activity 8.2 Visualisation for Grounding and Stabilisation: *The Exploding Volcano*

This active visualisation was created for clients who have already developed a sense of safety and rapport with the counsellor. It is not recommended for new clients.

This story could have lots of movement and noise in it. It is a story that can be acted out.

How do you feel about that? (pause for discussion).

This activity might help you have some fun, and then it could help you become peaceful. As I tell the story see how much you can imagine being in the story. See if you can make the sounds and the actions of everything in the story. Or, you might prefer to tell me about the sounds and movements?

Let's begin by standing up, stretching your body, running quickly on the spot for a moment, and taking a few deep breaths. Now, listen to what comes next:

This is a simple story, it is about a volcano. Picture yourself as an active volcano. This volcano is a mountain with hot lava, very hot melted rock, deep inside. There is a lot of smoke and steam rising up out of the top of you, into a cloud in the sky. Lava is rock deep under the ground and so hot it has turned bright red and melted, and can flow slowly, like super-hot melted chocolate.

From deep down below inside there is pressure building up from the molten rock, the lava. This lava is pushing up, it wants to escape. It is pushing up against a plug of solid rock at the top. The pressure is growing inside as the lava is pushing up. I think there could be a big release soon.

See if you would like to take a position that helps you feel a bit like the volcano, about to erupt. Maybe you could act out the pressure inside the volcano, show this with your hands, and with all your muscles.

You are the lava pushing up, and pushing up.

Suddenly the lava shoots up with lots of colours and sounds, and smoke and steam. The lava is bright and hot and flares up in all directions. Clouds of smoke and steam fill the sky.

See if you can imagine you are the orange and red lava, you are flowing down the side of the volcano.

As this liquid rock cools, it begins to flow more slowly. Your movement becomes slow. As the air cools, the rock stops still. And soon it is as still as stone.

See if you could be still like solid stone for a moment. Feel yourself breathing after the eruption. Now the volcano is peaceful again. The pressure has gone.

When you are ready to finish, you might like to draw something to remind you of how it felt to imagine or play out this story.

You might like to think about – and talk about – any times when you have felt similar to a volcano, and what happened then.

OPENING UP AND SHARING EXPERIENCES

Activity 8.3 Worksheet Reflection Activity: *Before I Talk about Myself …*

Materials: Worksheet *Before I talk about myself* (see Fig 8.1, page 212), crayons, pen, miniatures.

Aim: This activity is designed to help prepare clients to talk about self, gathering what they need to say, primarily for those clients who may not have an affinity with writing or using words. If your client is not keen to write, the activity could be used without words, using only symbols and colours and lines. Emphasise that there is choice in what they discuss.

Instructions

1. *On the worksheet, read through the sentence starters on the left. Find the prompt that seems interesting to you. Take some time to read it through.*
2. *With the words in that prompt in mind, see if you can find a symbol (or two) that goes with the words; and arrange these in the space on the worksheet.*
3. *Think about the symbols you have selected, then:*
   - *See if you would like to add some colours and lines to the space on the worksheet, something that helps show the mood or energies of the symbols or how they are connected or not connected with each other.*
   - *Next, could you find some words that go with the symbol(s)?*
4. *Take your time to work with any of the other prompts that are of interest to you.*
5. *Look over what you have created:*
   - *Does anything stand out to you?*
   - *Are there symbols you notice the most?*
   - *Are there colours, lines or words you notice most?*
6. *Could you put a tick or star beside whatever is most interesting on the worksheet.*
7. *When you are ready, see if you could say a little about how it felt to do the activity, and share anything that is important to you.*
8. *Is there anything you would want to say about the sentence starters not used?*

Worksheet: *Before I Talk About Myself . . .*	
Prompts and Starter Words	**Symbols, Colours, and Lines**
Friends . . .	
I think a lot about . . .	
Things I am really good at . . .	
If I could change anything . . .	

Figure 8.1 Worksheet – before I talk about myself.

9. *Would you be willing to sketch the symbols onto the page? Or photograph them?*

Suggestions for Prompts for Reflection – See Worksheet:

- *Friends …*
- *I think a lot about …*
- *Things I am really good at …*
- *If I could change anything …*

Further Suggestions for Prompts for Reflection:

- *My best strengths are …*
- *I don't want anyone to make me …*
- *I feel I need help with …*
- *I hope counsellors are good at …* (see Figure 8.1).

Activity 8.4 Self Esteem Worksheet: *My Best Quality, My Strength*

Suggested Age Range: From 12 years.

Materials: Art paper, crayons, journal, pen, worksheet: *My Best Quality, My Strength (Fig 8.2)*

Aim: To provide reflection and reinforcement on strengths and positive qualities.

- Invite the client to discuss what they think might be people's strengths and positive qualities. Are there any famous people they can think of who have strengths and positive qualities?
- Invite them to sit or lean back comfortably and take a few slow, full breaths. If they feel comfortable, invite them for a moment to close their eyes or soften their eyelids to support tuning in to self. Allow time to reflect, express and discuss each stage before moving on.

Identifying strengths: *Can you take a deep breath and relax it out? Reflect on what you think may be your best quality. What quality is your greatest strength?* (pause) *Can you tell me about it?*

Invite the client to discuss their strength(s).

1. **Somatic Location of Strengths**: *Can you relax again, and take another deep breath, and turn your focus to your body? Can you sense your best qualities and strengths in your body? Where would it live inside you? For example, would it be in your chest, legs, back, head, etc.?*

If you get a sense of where the best quality might be in your body, tune into it for a moment, then find a way to draw it onto the body outline on the worksheet.

2. **Colours, Lines and Shapes**: *Relax again, lean back, tune in. What would this quality look like if you could see it?*

What colours, lines or shapes would go with the quality, the strength you have found? It could be a picture of something from nature, like a plant or an animal, bird or fish, or simply lines and shapes.

Take a moment, and if something comes to your mind, see if you could do a sketch of that in the rectangle on the worksheet?

3. **Words**: *Tune into yourself again. Let your body relax as much as it can. Take a slow full breath. Tune into that body area again, connect with that quality, that strength.* (pause)

What words would be said, what phrases, statements would be made by this quality? If it could speak, what would it say? Are there any questions it would ask? (pause)

Would there be a name for this quality? Does it have a name? Could you write that?

Take time to write any words that come to you on the lines on your worksheet – in Step 3.

4. **Discussion**: The client is invited to talk about Steps 2 to 4.
5. **Visualise Expansion**: *When you are ready, can you relax again, tune in, and maybe close your eyes? Rest for a moment. Take time to breathe and be with the energy of this quality.* (pause)

See if you could imagine this strength expanding – as if you could let it grow with each breath. (pause).

Feel and imagine what it would be like inside if this strength extended all through you. Take a moment to picture this best quality growing.

Perhaps it could flow out into the world and express itself more often?

6. **Mandala Consolidation**:

When you are ready, see if you could create – in the mandala circle on your worksheet – something that goes with how you feel now? What colours, lines or pictures would go with this strength if it expanded all through you, and was able to express itself freely?

7. **Integration**: Invite the client to discuss what they have expressed on the worksheet and in the mandala;

   - how they felt during the activity and anything that stands out from the activity
   - what this quality brings to their life
   - is there anything it wants to create?

The client may also wish to focus on one particular segment and discuss it in more detail.

9. **Review the Sections of the Worksheet**:

- *Is there a statement you could make about how you can connect with this quality more in your life?*
- *How could it come out more?*

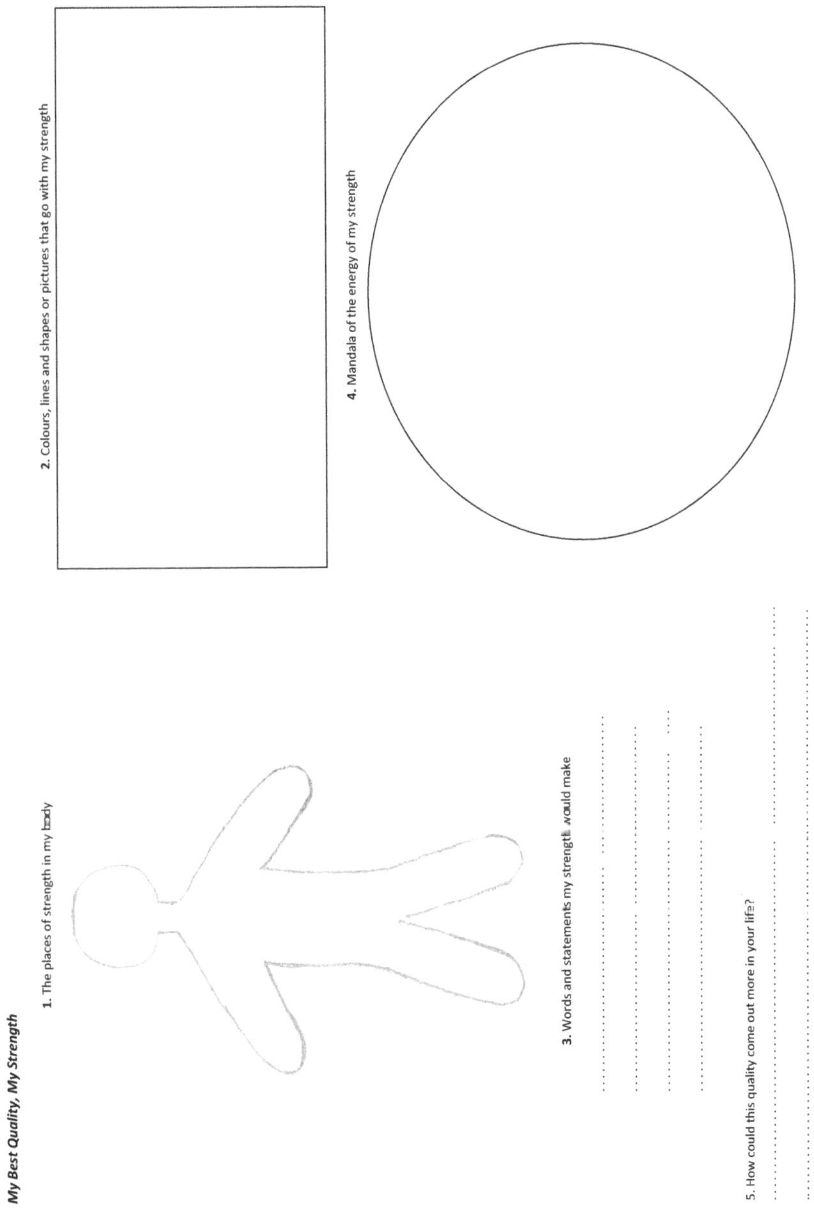

Figure 8.2 Worksheet – my best quality.

- *Could you write that on the worksheet?*
- *This could be a message from yourself to yourself.*
- *Would you like to share it?* (see Figure 8.2).

Activity 8.5 Safe Place Visualisation: *Time Out – My Connections to Nature*

Materials: Drawing paper, crayons, writing paper, pen.

Aim: To provide imagery of a safe place that can be used for psychological retreat from discomfort, when stress threatens to overwhelm the client – within or beyond the counselling session.

Part A

- Provide an overview of the activity.
- Invite the client to: *Tune-in, take a deep breath, see if you can remember or imagine* a *beautiful, safe area in nature that attracts you, a place you love to be, a place with some beauty, where you feel safe and happy.*

It could be a favourite beach, in the mountains, by a creek, or in a park, or

- *it may be a place where you can see the sky, trees, flowers, beautiful views*
- *it could be a special part of your garden at home or at a friend's place.*

- *Would you be willing to share what came to mind?*
- *Could you tune in again for a moment, take another deep breath, and imagine being back at this beautiful place in nature.*
  What are the main things you would see? Imagine looking up, down, from side to side.
  What would you see? hear? smell? touch?
  What would be the main feelings in you while you were in this place?
- *See if you could imagine moving through this place:*
  - *Become interested in the detail of what you remember, what you see in your mind.*
  - *Is there anyone there with you?*
  - *Take time and allow the pictures to soak in; enjoy them.* (pause)
  - *What stands out for you? Is there anything that is most noticeable in this place?*
- *When you are ready, move to the art paper and see if you could create a quick sketch of the main things you remember, or some parts of that beautiful place. It could be the whole place, or just a part of it. It does not matter if you are good at drawing or not. Simply sketch, as quickly as you can, something that will remind you of the place.*
- *If it helps, you could write down a few words about this place in nature. Perhaps you could give your sketch a title?*
- *Would you like to say a little about:*

- *What you created?*
- *The times you have been there? The sights, sounds, smells?*
- *If anyone was there with you?*
- *How did you feel being there?*

- Introduce the plan to use the image and memory of this place to "come back to" if they feel highly stressed in the counselling session or beyond. Both the client and the counsellor might suggest a re-visit at times, until the client's stress levels have decreased.

Part B

The counsellor offers an overview of the role-play, then invites the client to participate by asking the nine questions slowly. Give the client time to reflect and feel the answer, and then respond to your question. Make it clear they are also welcome not to respond.

- Say to the client:
- *Relax as much as you can and take a few deep breaths.*
- *For this activity, can you pretend you are this beautiful safe place in nature?*
- *And I will ask it – the space – some questions.*
- *You may like to close your eyes for a moment to help you imagine you are in a beautiful place.*
- *If you are comfortable to do so, allow a picture of the place to come into your mind's eye.*
- *Be interested in how it looks, feels and what its energy might be like.*
- *Now imagine you are becoming this beautiful place, with all its sights, sounds, colours.*
- *Take another full breath and feel how it is to be this beautiful safe place.*
- The client imagines self as the place in nature, then is invited to respond to these questions as the place, responding with *"I"* rather than *"It"*.

1. *Can you tell me what you are?*
2. *Would you be able to tell me what you look like?*
3. *Could you tell me about your atmosphere, mood or feelings?*
4. *What could you say about your age? Would you be old or young?*
5. *Can you tell me any ways you are safe, and any ways you are strong?*
6. *Do you have any sounds or movements? Could you show these?*
7. *Are there any ways you could help* ....(client's name)?
8. *Is there anything you want or hope for?*
9. *Do you have a message for* ....(client's name), *or anything you would like to say to him/her?* (pause) *Any advice perhaps? Or encouragement?*

After a pause say:

- *Now come back to being yourself, the person.*
- *Did you hear that message? How do you feel about that?*

- After some discussion, encourage the client to write down the message on the sketch of the safe place in nature.
- Invite the client to share how they feel after the activity and to share any ideas they have about the activity.

Somatic Connection: Reinforce the possibility to psychologically return to this place, when they feel highly stressed in life, or in the counselling session.

The place could be linked in their memory to an area in their body – such as the head, chest or belly. Ask them: *If the feeling of this place could be inside you, where would it be?* Take a moment for them to focus on the image and body area at the same time, to deepen the connection. Consider any times or places when this connection would be helpful. Invite the client to use the sketch as a reminder.

Activity 8.6 Timeline Worksheet: *Thinking about My Life*

Suggested Age Range: From approx. 13 to 19 years (also suitable for adults with minor column title adjustments).

Materials: A3 size *Life Review Time-Line* worksheet (Fig 8.3), crayons, miniatures, pen, *Feeling Words Lists* (see page 254).

Aims: Opens conversation about the client's life. Introduces the concept of reflection on, and review of, the past and future, and helps put events into sequence. Identify any life events or changes that (1) may need to be processed, (2) might hinder or assist a client's recovery from trauma.

Using the Worksheet:

- Ideally, the client works down each column, processing one stage of life at a time, saving the last section of each column until the end.
- Some clients may wish to reflect and fill out the worksheet with little discussion; others may wish to discuss each step.
- If there is a section that evokes no response, invite the client to simply move on to the next.

Read through the directions on the worksheet and clarify their meaning with the client.

Steps for Each Column:

1. *Colours and lines* for feelings that go with their memory of the stage of life.
2. Allow *images* to come to mind – and reflect these in the second rectangle of the column, *and/or select 1 or 2 miniatures* that remind them of this time – and place these in the rectangle.
3. Invite the client to recall any *major events* and their age at that time. Mark these on the time-line arrow.

Life Review Time-Line

BABY	TODDLER	CHILD	TEENAGER	FUTURE
Colours for the mood of this stage:	Colours for the mood of this stage:	Colours for the mood of this stage:	Colours for the mood of this stage:	Colours for my future mood:
1 or 2 symbols for this stage:	1 or 2 symbols for this stage:	1 or 2 symbols for this stage:	1 or 2 symbols for this stage:	1 or 2 symbols for your future:

Note major events on this time line:

Words for how this stage felt:	Words for how this stage felt:	Words for how this stage felt:	Words for how this stage felt:	What I would like is . . .
What stands out from this stage:	What stands out from this stage:	What stands out from this stage:	What stands out from this stage:	How I would like feel in the future:

Figure 8.3 Worksheet – life review time-line.

4. Find a few words for the *feelings of that time* – write these on the three lines. *The Feeling Words Lists* may help.
5. Invite the client to reflect on anything that stands out to them or has had an *impact* on their life then and now. Some discussion may be necessary before a summary is noted on the worksheet.

Discussion

- Are there any areas of the worksheet that stand out as being most interesting or emotionally charged for the client?
- Can these be attended to in more detail? e.g., through discussion, writing, addition of miniatures or moving into emotion-focused processes?
- Focus on the 5th column, the future – invite dreaming of *"What's next?"*

Integration

- Invite the client to discuss how they feel after completing and discussing the worksheet.
- What would they most like to remember from this activity? Are there any steps or directions or help in relation to the future?
- It may be helpful for the client to create an image of how they feel after completing the worksheet. This could be done in a circle (mandala) shape.
- The client may want to take a photograph of the completed worksheet. (Check safety of taking the image home) (see Figure 8.3).

References

American Psychological Association. (n.d.). Resilience. https://www.apa.org/topics/resilience/index

Asay, T. P., & Lambert, M. J. (1999). The empirical case for the common factors in therapy: Quantitative findings. In M. A. Hubble, B. L. Duncan, & S. D. Miller (Eds.), *The heart and soul of change: What works in therapy* (pp. 23–55). American Psychological Association.

Au, T. M., Sauer-Zavala, S., King, M. W., Petrocchi, N., Barlow, D. H., & Litz, B. T. (2016). Compassion-Based Therapy for trauma-related shame and posttraumatic stress: Initial evaluation using a multiple baseline design. *Behavior Therapy*, *48*(2), 207–221. https://doi.org/10.1016/j.beth.2016.11.012

Baloche, L. (1996). Clues about motivation and creativity. *Cooperative Learning*, *16*(3), 13–16.

Bartholomew, T. T., Joy, E. E., & Gundel, B. E. (2021). Clients' hope for counseling as a predictor of outcome in psychotherapy. *The Counseling Psychologist*, *49*(8), 1126–1146. https://doi.org/10.1177/00110000211033255

Barton, S., Gonzalez, R., & Tomlinson, P. (2012). *Therapeutic residential childcare for children and young people: An attachment and trauma-informed model for practice.* Jessica Kingsley Publishers.

Binda, D. D., Greco, C. M., & Morone, N. E. (2022). What are adverse events in mindfulness meditation? *Global Advances in Health Medicine, 19*(11), 2164957X221096640. https://doi.org/10.1177/2164957X221096640

Bolger, K. E., & Patterson, C. J. (2003). Sequelae of child maltreatment: Vulnerability and resilience. In S. S. Luthar (Ed.), *Resilience and vulnerability: Adaptation in the context of childhood adversities* (pp. 156–181). Cambridge University Press.

Cameron, R. J., & Maginn, C. (2009). *Achieving positive outcomes for children and young people in public care.* Sage.

Carey, L. J. (2006). *Expressive and creative arts methods for trauma survivors.* Jessica Kingsley Publishers.

Chafouleas, S. M., Johnson, A. H., Overstreet, S., & Santos, N. M. (2016). Toward a blueprint for trauma-informed service delivery in schools. *School Mental Health: A Multidisciplinary Research and Practice Journal, 8*(1), 144–162.

Clay, J. Z., Kane, S. J., & Zabelina, D. L. (2024). A brief online mindfulness induction improves creative art-making. *Psychological Research, 88*(1), 116–126.

Coholic, D., Lougheed, S., & Lebreton, J. (2009). The helpfulness of holistic arts-based group work with children living in foster care. *Social Work with Groups, 32*(29), 29–46. https://doi.org/10.1080/01609510802290966

Cooper, M. (2016). The fully functioning society: A humanistic–existential vision of an actualizing, socially just future. *Journal of Humanistic Psychology, 56*(6), 581–594.

Doyle, C. (2003). Child emotional abuse: The role of educational professionals. *Educational and Child Psychology, 20*(1), 8–21.

Duncan, B. (2010). On becoming a better therapist. *Psychotherapy in Australia, 16*(4), 42–51.

Feder, A., Nestler, E. J., & Charney, D. S. (2009). Psychobiology and molecular genetics of resilience. *Nature Reviews Neuroscience, 10*(6), 446–457.

Fredrickson, B. L., Tugade, M. M., Waugh, C. E., & Larkin, G. R. (2003). What good are positive emotions in crisis? A prospective study of resilience and emotions following the terrorist attacks on the United States on September 11th, 2001. *Journal of Personality and Social Psychology, 84*(2), 365–376.

Gallo, L. C., Penedo, F. J., Espinosa de los Monteros, K., & Arguelles, W. (2009). Resiliency in the face of disadvantage: Do Hispanic cultural characteristics protect health outcomes? *Journal of Personality, 77*(6), 1707–1746.

Gardner, H. (2006). *Multiple intelligences. New horizons.* Basic Books.

Garrett, K. E. (2020). Creative therapies, complex childhood trauma, and neurological improvement: How the arts can enhance neuroplasticity: A literature review. *Expressive Therapies Capstone Theses. 366.*

Germer, C. K. (2005). What is it? What does it matter. In C. K. Germer, R. D. Siegel, & P. R. Fulton (Eds.), *Mindfulness and psychotherapy* (pp. 3–27). Guilford.

Graber, R., Pichon, F., & Carabine, E. (2015). *Psychological resilience* (pp. 3–27). Overseas Development Institute.

Greenberg, L. S. (2002). Integrating an emotion-focused approach to treatment into psychotherapy integration. *Journal of Psychotherapy Integration, 12*(2), 154–189.

Greenberg, L. (2006). Emotion-focused therapy: A synopsis. *Journal of Contemporary Psychotherapy, 36,* 87–93.

Grepmair, L., Mitterlehner, F., Loew, T., & Nickel, M. (2007). Promotion of mindfulness in psychotherapists in training: Preliminary study. *European Psychiatry, 22*(8), 485–489. https://doi.org/10.1016/j.eurpsy.2007.02.004

Herman, J. (2015). *Trauma and recovery: The aftermath of violence – From domestic abuse to political terror.* Basic Books/Hachette Book Group.
Hinterkopf, E. (1998). *Integrating spirituality in counseling: A manual for using the experiential focusing method.* American Counseling Association.
Howe, D. (2005). *Child abuse and neglect: Attachment, development and intervention.* Palgrave Macmillan.
Hubble, M. A., & Miller, S. D. (2004). The client: Psychotherapy's missing link for promoting a positive psychology. In P. A. Linley & S. Joseph (Eds.), *Positive psychology in practice* (pp. 335–353). Wiley.
Jacobson, J. L. (2002). *An exploratory study regarding the effects of praying for others on physical and mental health in older adults* (Doctoral dissertation). Spalding University.
Jaaniste, J., & Perry, S. (2021). Art and dramatherapists together consider a multimodal approach for supporting clients with complex trauma. *JoCAT, 16*(1), 44–54.
Kabat-Zinn, J. (1994). *Wherever you go, there you are: Mindfulness meditation in everyday life.* Hyperion.
King, G. A. (2004). The meaning of life experiences: Application of a meta-model to rehabilitation sciences and services. *American Journal of Orthopsychiatry, 74*(1), 72–88.
Lambert, M. J. (1992). Implications of outcome research for psychotherapy integration. In J. C. Norcross & M. R. Goldstein (Eds.), *Handbook of psychotherapy integration* (pp. 94–129). Basic Books.
Lambert, M. J. (2005). Early response in psychotherapy: Further evidence for the importance of common factors rather than "placebo effects". *Journal of Clinical Psychology, 61*(7), 855–869.
Lightsey Jr, O. R. (2006). Resilience, meaning, and well-being. *The Counseling Psychologist, 34*(1), 96–107. https://doi.org/10.1177/0011000005282369
Lindsey, L., Robertson, P., & Lindsey, B. (2018). Expressive Arts and Mindfulness: Aiding Adolescents in Understanding and Managing Their Stress. *Journal of Creativity in Mental Health, 13*(3), 288–297. https://doi.org/10.1080/15401383.2018.1427167
Mace, C. (2007). Mindfulness in psychotherapy: An introduction. *Advances in Psychiatric Treatment, 13*(2), 147–154.
Malchiodi, C. (2020). *Trauma and expressive arts therapy. Brain, body, and imagination in the healing process.* The Guilford Press.
Marsh, C. (2003). A psycho-physiological comparison of post-traumatic and prolonged duress stress disorders. *Behavioural and Cognitive Psychotherapy, 31*(1), 109–112.
Masten, A. S. (2001). Ordinary magic: Resilience processes in development. *American Psychologist, 56*(3), 227–238. https://doi.org/10.1037/0003-066X.56.3.227
McLeod, J. (2018). *Pluralistic therapy: Distinctive features.* Routledge.
Mearns, D., & Thorne, B. (2000). *Person-centred therapy today: New frontiers in theory and practice.* Sage Publications.
Menninger, K. (1959). The academic lecture: Hope. *American Journal of Psychiatry, 116*(6), 481–491.
Monk, G. E., Winslade, J. E., Crocket, K. E., & Epston, D. E. (1997). *Narrative therapy in practice: The archaeology of hope.* Jossey-Bass.
O'Hara, D. (2025). Hope-focused therapy: A framework outline. *Psychotherapy and Counselling Journal of Australia*, 12(3), 45–60.

Oliver, K. G., Collin, P., Burns, J., & Nicholas, J. (2006). Building resilience in young people through meaningful participation. *Australian e-Journal for the Advancement of Mental Health, 5*(1), 34–40.

Pearson, M. (2011). Multiple intelligences and the therapeutic alliance: Incorporating multiple intelligence theory and practice in counselling. *European Journal of Psychotherapy & Counselling, 13*(3), 263–278.

Pearson, M., & Wilson, H. (2009). *Using expressive arts to work with mind, body and emotion. Theory and practice.* Jessica Kingsley.

Perry, B. D. (2006). Applying principles of neurodevelopment to clinical work with maltreated and traumatized children: The Neurosequential Model of Therapeutics. In N. B. Webb (Ed.), *Working with traumatized youth in child welfare* (pp. 27–52). The Guilford Press.

Perry-Parrish, C., Copeland-Linder, N., Webb, L., & Sibinga, E. M. (2016). Mindfulness-based approaches for children and youth. *Current Problems in Pediatric and Adolescent Health Care, 46*(6), 172–178.

Pynoos, R. S., Steinberg, A. M., Layne, C. M., Briggs, E. C., Ostrowski, S. A., & Fairbank, J. A. (2009). DSM-V PTSD diagnostic criteria for children and adolescents: A developmental perspective and recommendations. *Journal of Traumatic Stress, 22*(5), 391–398.

Rak, C. F., & Patterson, L. E. (1996). Promoting resilience in at-risk children. *Journal of Counseling & Development, 74*(4), 368–373.

Rempel, K. (2012). Mindfulness for children and youth: A review of the literature with an argument for school based implementation. *Canadian Journal of Counselling and Psychotherapy, 46*(3), 201–220. https://cjc-rcc.ucalgary.ca/article/view/59860

Rogers, C. R. (1951). *Client centered therapy. Its current practice, implications and theory.* Constable.

Rogers, C. R. (1980). Growing old–or older and growing. *Journal of Humanistic Psychology, 20*(4), 5–16. https://doi.org/10.1177/002216788002000403

Rothschild, B. (2010). *The body remembers. The psychophysiology of trauma and trauma treatment.* W. W. Norton & Company.

Scott, M. J., & Stradling, S. G. (1994). Post-traumatic stress disorder without the trauma. *British Journal of Clinical Psychology, 33*(1), 71–74.

Seewald, A., & Rief, W. (2024). Therapist's warmth and competence increased positive outcome expectations and alliance in an analogue experiment. *Psychotherapy Research, 34*(5), 663–678.

Schiffer, F., Teicher, M. H., & Papanicolaou, A. C. (1995). Evoked potential evidence for right brain activity during the recall of traumatic memories. *The Journal of Neuropsychiatry and Clinical Neurosciences, 7*(2), 169–175.

Siegel, D. J. (2007). *The mindful brain: Reflection and attunement in the cultivation of well-being.* WW Norton & Company.

Snyder, C. R., Michael, S. T., & Cheavens, J. S. (1999). Hope as a psychotherapeutic foundation of common factors, placebos, and expectancies. In M. A. Hubble, B. L. Duncan, & S. D. Miller (Eds.), *The heart and soul of change: What works in therapy* (pp. 179–200). American Psychological Association.

Sosin, L. S., Noble, S. D., Harrichand, J. J. S., & Bohecker, L. (2022). The Creative Arts Personal Growth Group (CAPG): Transforming fear and shame. *The Journal for Specialists in Group Work, 47*(2), 151–167. https://doi.org/10.1080/01933922.2021.2000083

Steele, W., & Malchiodi, C. A. (2012). *Trauma-informed practices with children and adolescents*. Taylor & Francis.
Strand, M., & Stige, S. H. (2021). Combining mindfulness and compassion in the treatment of complex trauma–a theoretical exploration. *European Journal of Trauma & Dissociation*, *5*(3), 100217.
Schut, M. S. H. (1999). The dual process model of coping with bereavement: Rationale and description. *Death Studies*, *23*(3), 197–224.
Terr, L. (1994). *Unchained memories*. Basic Books.
van Westrhenen, N., Fritz, E., Oosthuizen, H., Lemont, S., Vermeer, A., & Kleber, R. J. (2017). Creative arts in psychotherapy treatment protocol for children after trauma. *The Arts in Psychotherapy*, *54*, 128–135.
Wu, G., Feder, A., Cohen, H., Kim, J. J., Calderon, S., Charney, D. S., & Mathé, A. A. (2013). Understanding resilience. *Frontiers in Behavioral Neuroscience*, *7*, Article 10.
Yalom, I. D. (2001). *The gift of therapy*. HarperCollins.

9 A Positive Sense of Self

Mindfulness, Self-Esteem and Spirituality

Developing a Sense of Self

Erikson (1968) considered adolescence as a time when the development of a sense of self was a primary task. Spiegel introduced the concept of a "sense of self" to the New York Psychoanalytic Society in 1959. Although writers use the term in relation to a felt sense, a somatic connection, more often it relates to having a sense of individual identity. The American Psychological Association defines sense of self as "an individual's feeling of identity, uniqueness, and self-direction" (https://dictionary.apa.org/sense-of-self). Carl Rogers (1951) identified three contributing components to the development of the sense of self: Self-image, self-esteem and the ideal self. Finding new images of self, connecting with esteem or strengths and wrestling with differences between an ideal self and a perceived self, establishing a positive, stronger sense of self, can all be supported well through psychotherapy generally, and through ET in particular.

What does it mean to support a client to develop a stronger sense of self, and why is this useful? An impaired, or under-developed sense of self may be a basis for poor choices and behaviours that indicate counselling support would be useful. To begin this section, it may be helpful to explore a catalogue of some of the major causes and predictors of an impaired sense of self observed by the authors with clients and their families.

An impaired sense of self may result from the earliest possible influences, for example, from abuse, neglect, household dysfunction and early attachment difficulties. Studies on the impact of adverse childhood experiences have shown a significant impact on health and mortality (Jiaa & Lubetkinb, 2020), on adult mental health, including the risk of depression and suicide (Merrick et al, 2017).

There are also generational influences, such as parental modelling of self-esteem. This can occur explicitly and implicitly. Parental disharmony, family disintegration, family and cultural differences, even a negative family culture, in which disrespect, negative treatment, or the "tall poppy" syndrome flourish, may impair a sense of self. Having a history of shocks, disappointments or unresolved emotion – that activate memories of previous similar negative

DOI: 10.4324/9781003671879-9

emotional experiences – can inhibit maturation and identity development. Shocks would include experiences of abuse that result in a well-documented legacy of developmental complications. Difficulties arising from socio-economic backgrounds characterised by struggle, having a disability, or being different can shape a less-than-strong sense of self. The way a young person is treated at school, for example bullying, negative reactions from teachers and peers, vindictiveness, being on the receiving end of put-downs, can all contribute to an impaired sense of self. General, prolonged, social or academic stress such as elevated social expectations placed on a young person and/or demands for superior achievement, along with ongoing situations where personal value is based solely on achievement, may weaken a sense of self.

A number of signs raise the alert of impaired or underdeveloped sense of self. Some of these relate to a chronically low level of self-esteem. While any one sign may not indicate a delay or impairment of a sense of self, a combination of several most likely will. A child or young person may exhibit reactivity: Either withdrawal or acting-out; they may have a short attention span; they may display low interest in self-care, low social or academic motivation; they may even give up trying and sink into depression. Young people with a low sense of self may have difficulty in relating. For example, in relating, a consistent display of need for positive "feedback". Internally there may be a negative bias that boils down to: *I'm not good enough!*

Other signs of low sense of self may include excessive or obsessive concern about external appearance or achievement, a chronic state of anxiety or agitation, self-harming, heightened sensitivity to feeling different. Loss of emotional resilience means increased feelings of vulnerability, as well as inability to problem solve. In addition, a "failure mentality" may influence behaviour towards social cues. The world may be viewed through a particular "lens" – or script – that interprets events and relationships as proving negative self-perceptions, negative self-evaluations.

First and foremost, support for activating a stronger sense of self involves experiences of acceptance. While a therapist can offer accurate facts and highlight differences between negative self-belief and fact, it can take some time for a client to acknowledge these differences. Working with a counsellor who is comfortable with and supports emotional expression has the advantage that some of the pain of previous experiences can be processed as a prelude to change in self-relating, beliefs and behaviours. The process may include exploring unresolved recent and past issues and possibly enable focus on an original source of the negative sense of self. It may be valuable to help a client externalise and process self-blame, if needed, to open the way to recognition of original causes.

A team approach to recovery of a stronger sense of self works best. If a counsellor can work with the client, the family and the school – the whole system – positive outcomes are more likely. Ongoing support from the system, such as counselling sessions, extra-therapeutic leisure activities, classroom support, social networks, as well as ongoing contact with a positive, stable, self-aware adult (Fosha, 2003) may all contribute to building or re-building a solid sense of self. This is not always possible, especially in fragmented family situations.

Self-Esteem

While self-esteem has been defined as a positive or negative attitude towards the self (Rosenberg, 1965), there remains an absence of a universal definition for self-esteem. Several writers commented on the confusion in terminology used in popular and academic papers. However, Butler and Gasson (2005) found themes in the literature that offer clarity in relation to notions about self:

1. the global over-arching view of self may be regarded as "self-concept";
2. the evaluative aspect relates to worth and "self-esteem";
3. the descriptive facets referring to characteristics available to an individual in defining self may be understood as "self-image";
4. a notion of competency in terms of how effective a person considers they will be in undertaking a task has been referred to as "self efficacy".

Self-esteem includes positive or negative evaluations about oneself. It is described as our opinion of ourselves. It is common to lack confidence from time to time, but low self-esteem means a person is unhappy or unsatisfied with themselves much of the time. While on the fourth step of Maslow's (1943) hierarchy of needs, i.e., fairly high above safety needs, the need for self-esteem is presented as if a gate, which may be open or closed, or a crucial rung on a large ladder, to self-actualisation. The need for self-esteem – the fourth step of Maslow's (1943) hierarchy of needs – is represented as the gateway, or crucial rung on a ladder, to self-actualisation.

Constantly critical of themselves, a person with low self-esteem typically tends to downplay or ignore their positive qualities. Young people with low self-esteem engage in self-perceptions that incline them to use negative words to describe themselves. Furthermore, their internal self-talk continues to be negative, critical and self-blaming. Over time, self-hate and underlying negative self-concept are likely to consolidate identity. A person with low self-esteem finds it hard to accept compliments. Emler (2001) argued that low self-esteem individuals are inclined to treat themselves badly and may receive undesirable treatment from others, but tend not to treat others harmfully. Individuals with high self-esteem feel quite positive about their characteristics and competencies, which can positively influence wellbeing. Low self-esteem can be linked, on the other hand, to emotional and behavioural problems (Arslan, 2016).

Parents play a key role in a child's development of self-esteem. Supportive and warm parental acts and positive family experiences play a significant role in shaping self-esteem in children and adolescents (Shaffer & Kipp, 2010). Several processes link parenting styles with the self-esteem of children and adolescents (Pinquart & Gerke, 2019):

- High parental warmth is associated with positive approval of the child, which promotes the child's self-approval.
- Parental interest and focus promote the development of competence and success in important aspects of the child's life which are sources of self-esteem.
- Parental support of a child's autonomy satisfies a basic human need.
- Parenting styles may also be affected by the self-esteem of the child as parents may find it easier to show authoritative parenting towards well-adjusted children. Authoritative parenting was found to be related to higher levels of self-esteem, while the reverse was found for authoritarian and neglectful parenting (Pinquart & Gerke, 2019).

Resilience and self-esteem appear to play a protective role in emotional and behavioural problems in psychologically maltreated individuals. This is highly relevant considering that, in 2012, the worldwide prevalence of psychological maltreatment of children was estimated at nearly 36% (Stoltenborgh, et al., 2012). In 2024 WHO estimated 6 in 10 children (60%) regularly suffer physical punishment and/or psychological violence. The overall estimated prevalence rates for studies using informants were 4 per 1,000 for sexual abuse and 3 per 1,000, respectively, for physical abuse and emotional abuse. (Stoltenborgh, et al, 2014).

It can take attention and daily practice to boost low self-esteem (Victorian Government's "Better Health" website). Most of the advice for popular consumption – on this and many other websites – on counteracting low self-esteem provides cognitive solutions, based on the assumption that if we just thought more logically things could change. Most of us know that this can work for a short while, but long-term, some level of processing negative emotion-laden memories and responses related to past experiences is needed for consolidated change. For some young clients, it may take time to work through an internalised conviction about being inadequate. While ET provides a wide range of emotion-focused activities, it also provides many ways young clients can reflect on and articulate strengths or positive qualities in themselves. Having reminders, or reinforcers, of positive qualities – for example, clear metaphors, sketches, photographs of empowering symbols – can support a healthier review of attitudes towards self.

Developing Resilience

Resilience has been discussed in Chapter 8. Research on resilience and children emerged in the 1980s and focused on personal qualities of resilient children (Luthar, Cicchetti & Becker, 2000). Some current constructs of resilience see it as a personal trait or attribute, and others see it as an ongoing process of development of the ability to make positive adjustments (Lightsey, 2006). In the realms of therapy, the construct of resilience is central. Due to a growth in the focus on resilience through therapy, we explore further on the topic and how counselling, and ET in particular, contributes.

Masten's (2001) analysis of resilience studies led to the identification of several factors associated with resilience: Connections to competent and caring adults, cognitive and self-regulation skills, positive views of self and motivation to be effective in the environment. Several elements of personality have also been identified that distinguish resilient children from those who may become overwhelmed by negative factors (Rak & Patterson, 1996). These considerations include:

- an active approach towards problem solving,
- an ability to gain others' positive attention,
- an optimistic view of their experiences,
- an ability to maintain a positive vision of a meaningful life,
- the ability to be alert and autonomous,
- a tendency to seek novel experiences, and
- a proactive perspective.

We have found ET to be an ideal approach that can address and support the development of these fundamentals.

High school students identified perseverance, determination, social competence, self-efficacy, problem-solving skills, reflectivity, autonomy and a sense of purpose as key ingredients in their own protective factors (McMahon, 2007), showing some parallels with what researchers have observed. The students also referred to self-esteem development as integral to their academic success.

There is little evidence that some children are simply resilient by nature; either somewhere in the child's background is supportive care, or during the time of recovery there has been extra support (Weinfield, et al., 1999). Professional counsellors can make a significant contribution to supportive care. Children with secure histories are more resistant to stress and more likely to rebound following a period of troubled behaviour (Weinfield, et al., 1999).

A sense of humour plays an important role in contributing to resilience (Earvolino-Ramirez, 2007). In making light of difficulties, coping mechanisms are enhanced and can decrease the intensity of emotional reactions. Humour has also been found to have a beneficial effect on health (Earvolino-Ramirez, 2007). Our experience is that adolescent clients have the ability to switch focus rapidly from serious and stressful topics to appreciating the humour in many human situations. While the use of humour has generally not been incorporated as part of the professional skills of counselling, encouraging clients' abilities to take a break from dealing with difficulties through humour could be part of a counsellor's role. And, of course, counsellors are more likely to be able to tap into this ability if they can find a similar attitude in themselves.

Meaning in life has been identified as a predictor of resilience and wellbeing (Lightsey, 2006). Increase meaning in life was found to predict a positive change in mental health (Jacobson, 2002). Several of the activities in this chapter are designed to support connection with meaning, initially in symbolic form. Meaning is established through belonging, doing and understanding (King, 2004). Counselling using ET processes supports these and offers multiple opportunities for "doing", for belonging, particularly in groupwork.

In ET practice, the communication and attachment style of the counsellor aims to be focused, attuned and caring, in some ways reflecting an ideal early parent-child connection. This echoes Rogers' (1951) emphasis on creating, in therapy, a relationship characterised by unconditional positive regard to support effective psychological change.

Positive emotions are active ingredients within resilience (Fredrickson et al., 2003). Findings suggest that positive emotions experienced after a crisis act as a buffer against depression, particularly in resilient individuals. Positive emotions, such as gratitude, interest, love, etc., were seen to support coping. Positive emotions put people's minds at ease, have the capacity to create relaxation in the body, and can lower heart rate and blood pressure (Fredrickson et al., 2003). Resilient people use imagery or memory to generate positive emotions for soothing (Greenberg, 2002). It has been noted that resilient people create positive emotions in themselves. This in turn brings forward positive emotions in others close to them. Recurring experiences of positive emotions within therapy support resilience building. These experiences are more likely to emerge after processing emotional distress and working through what lies at the foundation of an impaired sense of self.

ET in Resilience Development

Groupwork and group counselling provide resilience-building support through the potential to form new peer bonds. Facilitators of ET groupwork programmes report observations of these resilience-building capacities. The use of groups is recommended for the development of resiliency skills, along with the use of role-play and creative imagery. Outcomes include improved self-expression and broader conflict resolution techniques (Rak & Patterson, 1996).

We recommend that counsellors relate to clients from an underlying focus on reclaiming resourcefulness. Resilience can be enhanced through gaining a sense of satisfaction with their level of involvement in the therapeutic process. The positive assumptions that underlie a therapeutic relationship encourage a client's ability to work through issues and build resilience. Ideally, a therapist will relate to a client from an attitude of certainty that the client has the internal resources necessary to work through their issues. This leads to optimism and an experience of success. Success is one of the ingredients that builds resilience (Doyle, 2006).

Resilience researchers recommend avoiding a one-size-fits-all approach. The uniqueness of the client calls for creating interventions tailored to each specific client, depending on "gender, age, culture, risk exposure and access to protective resources" (Graber, et al., 2015, p. 17). Adoption of an integrative approach that respects individual differences and has the capacity to activate client resilience is likely to yield optimum outcomes.

Mindfulness

Mindfulness is "paying attention in a particular way: on purpose, in the present moment, and nonjudgmentally" (Kabat-Zinn, 1994, p. 4), and "awareness of present experience with acceptance" (Germer, 2005, p. 7). Mindfulness is a term being used more frequently in the therapeutic and psychological literature. Mindfulness has become popular among therapists, and its practice has implications for integration of the therapy process. Focusing attention internally can provide building blocks for new neural pathways (Siegel, 2007). Some degree of mindful focus is introduced in ET, in almost every session.

Promoting mindfulness in therapists has an influence on the treatment results of their clients (Grepmair et al., 2007). A short programme of mindfulness meditation produced observable effects on brain and immune function (Davidson et al., 2003), suggesting that meditation may change brain and immune function in positive ways. Most of us seeking to work with young people will be focusing on what we DO. What seems clear is that children learn most from modelling what we ARE. An important aspect of our preparation to support others is to experience our own therapeutic support, to clear any of our own reactivity, to come to a fuller connection with ourselves. Working towards supporting from a more mindful state provides a direct model for clients.

Introducing Mindfulness Activities

A Script to Help Young Clients

Becoming more aware of ourselves, becoming more mindful, can help us reduce stress and anxiety. There are many types of activities that invite us to become more focused, more mindful. Some use movement, some use imagination, some encourage stillness. Mindfulness practice is a time to pay attention, to focus, to get to know what is happening inside. While relaxation can bring feelings of warmth and softness, mindfulness can bring a sense of increased alertness.

Each day we spend so much time looking at, and listening to, everything around us. Sometimes we worry about what others think about us, what happened yesterday, what might happen next. We can get so used to worrying. Mindfulness gives us the time to look and listen inside us, to let go of the outside world and our worries for a moment, and notice what is happening right now.

Why Is It a Good Idea to Practice Mindfulness?

As we practise mindfulness, we increase our capacity to concentrate; we may worry less. We may be helped by letting go of very high expectations of ourselves. Mindfulness can help us feel calmer and think more clearly.

Mindfulness can seem difficult. We may try to be quiet and still, and at the same time notice that we have busy thoughts. We may realise we are listening to sounds around us and lose concentration. Learning mindfulness can be frustrating at first. However, with practice, we can start to let go of worries, stresses and upsets. Usually, we can only pay attention to what is happening inside us for a short time. But that is what it is all about: The practice, how we learn to pay attention.

Sitting still, doing nothing, can feel uncomfortable. Mindfulness can help build confidence and a feeling of strength. Getting to know what is happening inside you is important in making decisions and understanding how we connect with others. There are many skills to learn through these activities: You can learn to become peaceful, to watch your thoughts and feelings without being swamped by them, and we learn to let the stress float away. Learning to concentrate will be very helpful for you throughout your whole life.

So, if you notice you are not listening, or thinking about yesterday or tomorrow, or wondering what people outside are saying or doing, all you have to do is take a deep breath, focus inside yourself and start to pay attention again. It does not matter how often you start again!

For meditation activities designed to help us feel more alert, more awake, it is usually best to do them sitting in a comfortable chair. Most people like to close their eyes when they want to focus, so they are not distracted by what is happening around them. Whether you sit in a chair or on a cushion, find a position where you can relax and still feel awake.

Making Space for Spirituality

Something that may be both a component of a positive sense of self and a pathway to establishing it is spirituality. Within therapeutic relating, we have encountered a shift at times in client focus and expression. This shift is towards sharing existential interests that contain a "spiritual" dimension. Since 2000, there has been a rapid growth of the literature on children's spirituality (Coholic, 2010). Seeking reconnection with and exploration of the importance of spirituality was noted by humanistic psychologists such as Maslow and Rogers, and by existential theorists Frankl and Fromm (Coholic, 2010).

Spirituality has been associated with emotional and behavioural health (e.g., Dragan et al., 2025; Vitorino et al., 2018). Research has supported the notion that spirituality has a positive impact on individuals' mental and physical health (Haug, 1998; Vitorino et al., 2018). For example, a systematic review of literature showed that 79% of studies of spirituality in mental health journals demonstrated benefits from spiritual practice (Sifers et al, 2012). Spiritual competency encompasses the ability to conceptualise and utilise a client's spiritual experience in clinical contexts, while remaining free from any bias through self-awareness and knowledge (Joslin & Gingrich, 2022).

Spirituality is an integral part of the study of humanity and resilience (Sifers et al., 2012). Research supports the beneficial role of spirituality for youth who are at risk for negative developmental outcomes. Spirituality and religion are also associated with thriving and lower rates of problem behaviours in youth who are not high-risk (Sifers et al., 2012). Spirituality can provide meaning for life and explanations for events, which may lead to a sense of comfort, hope and value in the face of the challenges of life (Haug, 1998).

Because of developmental limitations of children's language to articulate complex experiences, artistic expression has been a recommended way of accessing and exploring children's spirituality (Park, 2013). Art interventions had a positive, measurable effect on growth in spirituality and self-esteem in children who participated in eight weeks of sessions (Heer, 1998).

When supporting children through an impactful life event – such as trauma, grief, or loss – it is important to attend to their spiritual experiences, their perceptions and ways of knowing (Boynton & Mellan, 2021). In one study, children preferred spiritual dialogue and content to involve creativity, play and expression (Boynton, 2016). Part of children's spiritual expression includes the sacred, the fantastical, and the deep relational connections they have with others, with nature and/or a higher power (Boynton, 2016). Children have a distinct spiritual presentation often characterised by relationship, magical thinking and intuition (Cervantes & Arczynski, 2015). Some children naturally exhibit a sense of wonder, awe and curiosity about the natural world – something counsellors recognise as spiritual (Worthington et al., 2011). We have observed that connections with nature and with a higher power may emerge from young clients and become clarified and communicated through the visual art, symbol work and sandtray creations.

Counsellors working with play therapy were found to be interested in the symbolic expressions of spirituality of their young child clients (Worthington et al., 2011). The use of sandtray was common, and the data in Worthington et al.'s study demonstrated a link between sandtray work and children's spirituality. It was described as the *"best metaphor for spirituality because there are always symbols that are put in that are spiritual symbols"*. The same ability to express using symbols applies to ET symbol work.

Pandya (2024) found that spirituality can be linked to nurturing creativity among children. Times of spiritual reflection and expression bolster creativity in young people. This may have valuable implications for the future development of problem-solving skills. Spirituality, like the expressive arts, is largely about process rather than the created artefact. A dominant metaphor for spirituality is the "journey", which evokes a sense of constant movement and progression (Paintner, 2007). Recognising therapy as part of a journey, rather than a problem-focused emergency, can support a positive sense of self for clients who somehow interpret this need for therapy as a sign of weakness or deficiency.

A study that examined adolescents' understanding of spirituality and its relationship to resilience was conducted by Raftopoulos and Bates (2011). Three aspects of spirituality emerged: (1) a transcendental perspective expressed as a relationship with God or a higher power, (2) sense of meaning and (3) connection with the inner self. These dimensions fostered resilience by providing: (1) a sense of protection, comfort and security, (2) a sense of meaning, coherence and optimism and (3) the opportunity for increased self-awareness and self-efficacy. The broad aim of enhancing a client's "connection with the inner self" sits at the heart of the ET approach.

Some ET activities are designed to allow contact with self in a way that could be described as "deeper" than usual. Some provide a framework onto which clients can project their unique sense of spiritual questioning. While we never apply our own personal perspectives on spirituality, it is vital that activities, time and space be made for young clients to feel comfortable to explore questions about God, life, death, existence.

SELF-ESTEEM ACTIVITIES

Activity 9.1 Self-Esteem Role-Play: *My Treasure Revealed*

Suggested Age Range: From 10 years.

Materials: Crayons and A3-sized drawing paper (with clipboard).

Aim: To contribute to a revised view of self, an expanded sense of self.

Note: This activity is most successful when there is a beautiful view onto nature, some natural bush or a garden outside the consulting room. If not, prepare several scenes from nature that can be used as an alternative. The counsellor accompanies the client at all times.

Instructions

- *Take the paper on the clipboard and the crayons with you, then take time to look outside for a few minutes. Look around in all directions. What do you notice in the view? Look carefully at nature.*
- *What draws your attention? Is there something that stands out as most precious and special to you? It can be big, or it could be small. It could be up, it could be down. What – in nature – stands out as special?*
- *Look at it carefully, then sketch the special thing as best you can.*

Discussion

Return inside.

- *Can you think of a title for your sketch?*
- *Would you be willing to show your drawing and talk about what attracted you to what you have drawn?*
- *Can you close your eyes for a moment and pretend you are the thing you have drawn? Could you tell me:*
  - *What you are?*
  - *What you look like?*
  - *What your main feelings are at the moment?*
  - *About your sounds or movements?*
  - *What you are for, what you are doing there?*
  - *Do you have a message for* ....(client's name), *or anything you would like to say to him/her? Any advice perhaps? or encouragement?*

After a pause say:

- *Now come back to being yourself, and then gently open your eyes.*
- *Did you hear that message? How does that feel?*
- Can you write down the message.
- Invite them to share how they feel after the role-play, and to share any ideas about how it would be helpful to their life.

Activity 9.2 Visualisation, Drama and Drawing: *The Mysterious Island*

Suggested Age Range: From 9 years.

Materials: Drawing books and crayons ready.

Note: Suitable as an individual or group activity. It is ideal, but not essential, to flow into Part B, the role-play stage of the activity. The client can act out the story, or be still and visualise.

Aim: To provide a framework, via visualisation, for the client to build some connection to strength in self.

Part A: Visualisation – *The Journey to the Island*

- Client stands, stretches and takes some deep breaths.
- Explain the concept of a visualisation.
- Setting the scene for the visualisation:

This activity takes you on an imaginary journey to find a surprise. You could stand up and do some of the actions, or if you like, settle into a comfortable chair and let your mind do the work.

(Gentle drumming/rhythmic background music)

This is a time hundreds of years ago, a very, very long time ago. Imagine you and your tribe are beside the ocean. This is where you live. It is a simple life: you go swimming, fishing, playing. And life is very simple.

It is a warm, calm night. It is the full moon night and your tribe has gathered to celebrate beside the ocean. Everyone joins in the feasting, dancing and drumming. You dance on into the night. You are dancing around the fire with your tribe. The drums are playing. Everyone has enjoyed a great feast. This is a time for fun and celebration of life.

The full moon is high in the sky. The light of the moon is brightest on the beach and the ocean, and the moon is shining a silver path out across the water. The water is calm, with gentle waves.

The night is warm. The drums give you strength. You feel good, and strong.

A great idea pops into your head! And you want to take your canoe and set out on an adventure across the ocean.

See if you can imagine your canoe, a small boat for paddling over the water.

It is time to launch the canoe. You slide it down the beach, into the water, and set out over the waves. You have a paddle to push your boat through the water. You paddle out, following the moon's path. You paddle and paddle, but don't feel tired. You can hear the tribe a long way off in the distance. You can hear your canoe pushing through the water.

You have paddled long, and now notice daylight starting to glow orange and yellow on the horizon. Ahead, you can see the shape of a mysterious island.

You have never seen it before. You know that it is where you are meant to go. You paddle faster now! You paddle over the gentle waves, ashore to the island. You pull the canoe up the beach, and walk up the sand to the grass.

You look about and see a track through the jungle. You head towards the middle of the island through the trees, through the thick jungle. The track is there to guide you.

The track leads to the centre of the island, past the jungle, to an empty clearing in the middle of the island. Stand still now at the edge of the clearing.

As the morning light becomes stronger, you watch what's happening in the centre of the island.

Imagine you are in the centre of the island, watching and waiting. What can you discover there? Something will come into your imagination.

It will be a surprise, something wonderful, beautiful, something unexpected. See what is happening there, in the centre of the island, see every detail. Watch and wait for your imagination to show you this amazing surprise. I will be quiet for a moment now. (pause)

The day becomes brighter and hotter. Now it is time to return to your tribe, to your homeland. It is time to leave the surprise.

So, turn away now from the centre of the island. Carefully, you follow the track back towards the beach, past the jungle, across the grass, down the sandy beach.

You slide your canoe down the sand, back to the water, and paddle towards home.

Now, you start to see your beach, your homeland.

You are back on your beach now, back with your tribe. Could you sketch the surprise that you found in the centre of the island? People want to know what you saw. So, when you are ready, could you do a quick sketch of the surprise? (Pause while they draw.)

Could you write down something about the surprise?

- *What was it?*
- *What strengths does it have?*
- *In what ways is this surprise in the centre of the mysterious island a little bit like you?*

- Invite them to discuss what they saw.
- Use Part B the *Role-Play* (next) to explore the meaning of the surprise and to "hear" the message of what was going on at the centre of the island.

Part B: Role-Play – Understanding the Surprise on the Island

- The counsellor will invite comments about the surprise the client saw in the middle of the Mysterious Island (previous page), then invite them to role-play the image.
- Ask the following questions slowly, giving the client time to reflect and feel the answer, and then respond.
- Say to the client:
  - *Relax as much as you can and take a few deep breaths.*
  - *Can you pretend you are the surprise at the centre of the island?*
  - *Even if it sounds strange, could you try it? And I will ask it some questions.*
  - *If you are comfortable to do it, close your eyes for a moment, let a picture of the surprise come into your mind's eye.*
  - *Be interested in how it looks.*
  - *Now let yourself become this surprise.*
  - *Imagine your body changing; change the way you sit if it helps.*
  - *Feel the energy of this surprise – you are it now!*
  - *Take a full breath and feel how it is to be it. I am going to ask this surprise a few questions.*
- The client first imagines self as the surprise from the island then answers these questions, responding with *"I"* rather than *"It"*.

1. *Can you tell me what you are?*
2. *What is the most surprising thing about you?*
3. *Feel inside what you are made of, or what is inside you?*
4. *Can you tell me about your age? Are you old or young?*
5. *Do you have a sound or movement?*
   a. (If they do ask them to demonstrate it)
6. *Do you have any strong feelings?*
7. *Do you have a special purpose? What are you for?*
8. *Is there anything you want?*
9. *Do you have a message for* ....(client's name), *or anything you would like to say to him/her? Any advice perhaps? or encouragement?*

After a pause say:

- *Now come back to being yourself, and then gently open your eyes.*
- *Did you hear that message? How does that feel?*

- After some *discussion* encourage them to *write* down the message and the main qualities of the surprise.
- Invite them to share:
  - how they feel after the role-play
  - any ideas about how it relates to their life.

Activity 9.3 Self-Esteem Visualisation: *Inside Me Is the Very Best*

Suggested Age Range: From 9 years.

Materials: Drawing and writing materials ready. See also Part B *Role-Play of the Gift* – next page.

Aim: A visualisation activity to find images that represent positive qualities of self, inner resources, resilience, in symbolic form and explore and integrate these with role-play.

Note: For clients from 17 years to adult, modify the visualisation so that they are led to buy a present, or watch an exotic animal, bird or fish in the wild, or go to the best concert in the world.

Part A: Visualisation – *The Shopping Trip*
Explain what a visualisation is. Set the scene: Client will imagine themselves as extremely wealthy. Brief discussion on how that would feel.

Sit comfortably and relax. You can close your eyes if you wish, if it helps you imagine. Take some deep breaths, and relax as much as you can.

Imagine you are very, very wealthy. Very, very rich. So rich that you could do anything, go anywhere and buy absolutely anything in the world.

Sometimes you go shopping for gifts for your family, with your pockets full of money, sometimes you use a special Golden Credit Card, which has no limit.

You like to help others with your wealth. You are very generous. But, today you are taking time off. You are going on a shopping trip to buy something special for yourself – a wonderful gift just for you!

You have your own jet, of course. Imagine yourself now in your jet, in a big comfortable seat, sipping your favourite drink peacefully flying above the clouds.

Remember this is your day to go shopping for yourself.

See if you can imagine a special country where you want to go shopping.

What country would that be? Imagine this. Where would you most like to go shopping?

When you are ready, imagine asking the pilot to land your jet there.

You have a very fast jet, of course, so fast that your pilot is starting to land already. Look out the window. What do you see?

When you land you see that someone is waiting to take you to the shopping place. How do you go? In a car? a boat? a carriage? on horse-back? on a motor bike? Or do you simply walk?

Now you are walking down the street. See the shops. Are there buildings? Is it an open-air market place? Is it a city? See what comes into your mind.

Soon you become attracted to one shop. What sort of shop is it? What do they sell? Do you go inside? Imagine yourself walking about, looking at what is for sale there.

You are going to buy yourself a very beautiful, special gift, something of great quality. It could be something serious, it could be big or small. It could be a fun thing.

Check that you feel good buying something for yourself. Remember, you've helped others, and today it is your turn.

In your imagination, select what attracts you the most in the shop. It might be something you have always wanted – or it might be a complete surprise!

It could be anything! Remember, there is no limit! Wait and see what the gift will be. (pause)

Can you see the gift clearly in your mind? Look at every detail of it.

Expression

When you are ready, move to the paper and crayons. Could you sketch the gift you have selected for yourself? Even if you don't like to draw, quickly sketch something that will remind you of the gift.

Discussion

The client is invited to talk about:

- the gift, and what they might do with it
- how it felt to be rich
- the country they went to
- how it felt to buy the gift.

The gift you bought for yourself can show you some positive qualities about you – so get ready to hear about them! We are going to see if you can discover more about yourself.

Part B: ***Integration of the Gift***

- After the client has shared their experience of being wealthy, the travel and shopping and the gift, the counsellor will ask them to imagine becoming the gift, then answer the following questions. Give the client time to reflect, allow an answer to form and then respond.
- **Say to the Client**:
  - *Relax as much as you can and take a few deep breaths, feel the chair beneath you. Feel your breath coming and going.*
  - *Can you pretend you are this gift you brought for yourself?*
  - *I will ask the gift some questions, and you can let the gift answer.*
  - *If you are comfortable to do it, you can close your eyes for a moment and let a picture of the gift come into your mind's eye.*
  - *Be interested in how the gift looks and feels. See if the gift has a mood.*

- *Now let yourself become this gift.*
- *Imagine your body changing; change how you are sitting if it helps.*
- *Take some full breaths, and feel how it is to be the gift.*
- The *client imagines self as the gift* then answers these questions, ideally responding with *"I"* rather than *"It"*.

1. *Can you tell me what you are?*
2. *Would you be willing to describe what you look like?*
3. *Feel inside, could you tell me what you are made of, or what is inside you?*
4. *Do you have a special purpose? What are you for?*
5. *Can you tell me about your beauty and strengths?*
6. *How would this strength be helpful for* ....(client's name)?
7. *Is there anything you want for* ....(client's name)?
8. *Do you have a message for* ....(client's name), *or anything you would like to say to him/her/them? Any advice perhaps? or encouragement?*

After a pause say:

- *Now come back to being yourself, and slowly open your eyes. You are you now.*
- *Did you hear those messages? How does that feel?*

- After some discussion encourage them to repeat and reinforce the message, and write down the most important message beside the picture.
- Invite them to describe how they feel after the role-play and any insights about how the message relates to their life.

Activity 9.4 Self-esteem Worksheet: *My Journey from Problems to Treasure*

Suggested Age Range: From 10 years.

Materials: Worksheet – *My Journey from Problems to Treasure* (Fig 9.1, see page 244), coloured pencils or crayons, pen, private journal or writing paper, drawing paper, completion sentence-starters (see following activity). Symbols may also be useful.

Note: Recommended for later stages in the therapeutic process.

Aim: To develop language for communication and provide the client with a framework to reflect on their therapeutic journey, acknowledge positive aspects of self, and look to the future.

Instructions to Client:

This worksheet has been designed to help you explore some feelings, ideas, dreams and hopes from your inner world.

- *It can help you discover more about the feelings that go with any problems in your life, and the treasures and strengths inside you that may be hidden, or not thoroughly seen by others.*
- *Spend some time working through the three columns. You can keep the worksheet private or share what you discovered about yourself. You are free to say as much or as little about yourself as you wish. You can decide if you want to show your worksheet to anyone or keep it private, in the room here with me.*

Problems or Challenges:

Starting with the column headed "Problems and Challenges", take a moment to think about any problems.

- *Even if you haven't any clear ideas, maybe you have a feeling or memory inside you that seems like a problem.*
- *If you can't think of any problems, move on to the second column.*
- *Create in the first circle any colours, shapes, lines or pictures that somehow show how your problems feel to you.*
- *Next think about some words that might go with the problems or feelings and write these on the dotted lines under the circle.*
- *Next you are invited to think of any pictures from nature that are like your problems.*
- *For example, are your problems like a thunderstorm? an ocean? a desert? a jungle, like wild animals, like tiny ants? You could think about places close to nature you have been, or animals you have seen at the zoo or on TV.*

Treasure:

In the next column, you are invited to think about positive qualities, treasures or strengths inside you.

- *Could you find words that go with treasures that might be hidden within you?*
- *Next, are there any images from nature that go with these treasures? What comes to your mind? Some people like to think of gems, crystals, beautiful places, beautiful birds or animals.*
- *Then use colours and lines and shapes and pictures to express in the second circle how these treasures feel, or what they might look like.*

Future:
The third column looks towards the future.

- *Take a moment to close your eyes and reflect on the future generally, and particularly your own future.*
- *Watch in your mind's eye and see if any colours, lines or pictures emerge. Then create an image in the circle.*
- *Next find some words that might describe the feelings of your future. For example, would it feel: Good? dark? scary? bright? happy? etc.*
- *Then again, think about nature. Are there any pictures from nature that come to your mind that go with your future?*

Integration

Use these Sentence Starters:

- *Take time now to write down* (or discuss) *a summary by finishing these sentences:*
  - *The part I liked* ....
  - *The part I didn't like* ....
  - *The main strength or treasure inside me is* ....
  - *This could help me handle problems by* ....
  - *All the treasure inside me would make my future more* ....
  - *I now feel* ....

Discussion

Is there anything that stood out, or seemed most important to you from the worksheet or the sentences?

- *What parts of the worksheet seemed most important to you?*
- *How did you feel doing the worksheet?*
- *Were there parts of the activity you didn't like?*
- *Do you think you made any discoveries about yourself?*
- *Can you say anything more about the future?*

- Ask the client what they would like to do with the worksheet (see Figure 9.1).

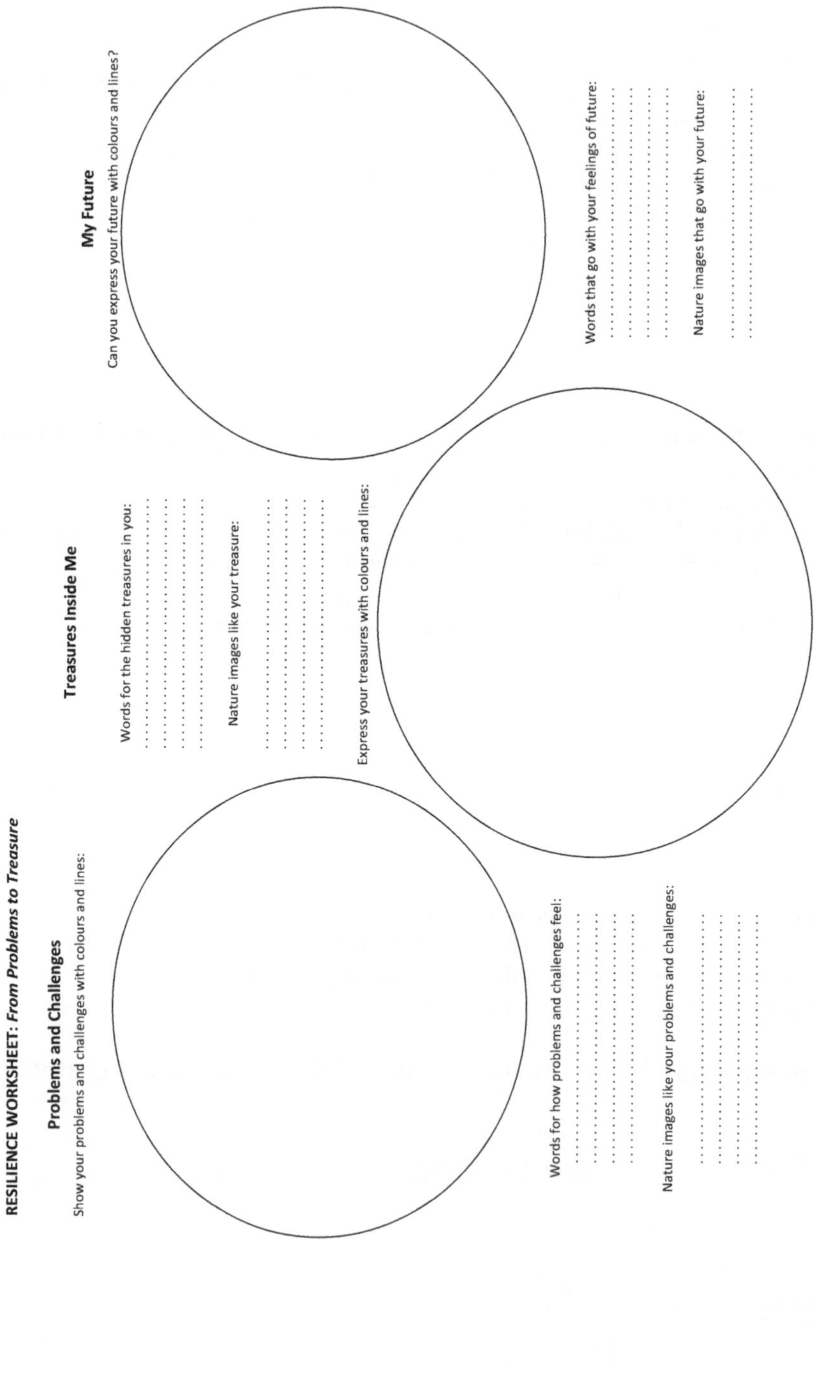

Figure 9.1 Worksheet – problems to treasure.

ACTIVITIES TO INTRODUCE MINDFULNESS

Activity 9.5 Visualisation for Relaxation: *An Iceberg Melts*

Age Range: From 6 or 7 years.
Materials: Paper and crayons.

Instructions

- *Lean back, relax, close your eyes if you like. Take three big slow breaths, and relax them out.*
- *Imagine yourself as an iceberg floating in the icy ocean near the South Pole. It is very cold there. An iceberg is a huge chunk of ice, sometimes as big as a city building, floating in the ocean. It is usually very big, with just its tip rising above the water. Imagine you are the iceberg now. You are moved by the wind and water currents.* (pause)
- *You are floating towards the warm climates. In tropical climates, it is very warm, and this is where you are heading, away from the cold and ice. There are palm trees and beautiful beaches. The sun becomes very hot. The sun shines down now on that part of you that is above the water. And the ocean is warming up too! So there is warmth above you and warmth below.*
- *You know what happens when ice warms up. What happens as you – the iceberg – start to melt? What does it feel like to join up with the ocean, to be part of the ocean? Imagine yourself joining with the ocean. Imagine that the water in you, that was frozen, is becoming warm and blending in with the whole ocean. The sun is hot, the air is warm, the water is warm. Imagine yourself being part of the ocean, flowing with the warm ocean current.* (pause)
- *Has all the hard ice melted yet? Are there any frozen parts left?*
- *Check if your arms are warm and melted. Tune in to your legs, are they warm and melted? How does it feel in the middle of your body? Can you imagine the middle of your body becoming warm, melting and floating with the ocean current?*
- *See if you can stay like that for a while.* (pause)
- *Imagine all of you are warm and flowing now, floating gently with the ocean, towards the warm tropics, moving freely to new lands, being carried by the warm water.*
- *Now slowly take a breath, move a little, move your toes, your fingers. When you are ready, let your eyes open and, when you are ready, come back to being you, here in this room now.*

Students are invited to draw what it felt like to be floating in the warm ocean.

Discussion:

- *How do you feel now?*
- *How did you feel before the exercise?*

- *Are there any parts that took longer to melt?*
- *Can you think of any times when it would be useful to feel relaxed?*

Activity 9.6 Somatic Awareness Activity: *Visualising Relaxation*

Age Range: From 8 to 9 years.
Materials: Paper and crayons.

- Uses both physical relaxation and visualisation to assist the body to let go and come to a quiet state.
- Client is invited to relax their back on a carpeted floor.

Instructions

(Give Instructions Slowly)

- *Take a moment to relax your whole body as much as you can. Let it go floppy. Close your eyes.*
- *Become aware of your neck. Imagine your neck is becoming floppy – and growing longer.*
- *Let the middle of your body be free, imagine it becoming softer, melting. Picture this happening. Imagine or think it.*
- *Become aware of your chest. Give your chest permission to let go now, to melt down, to be like cheese on a hot pizza. Tune in to the space between your shoulders now.*
- *Imagine your shoulders widening a little. Allow your body to follow this image.*
- *Tune into your belly. Is anything tight? Could you relax more in your belly, like a kitten asleep by a warm fire?*
- *Move your focus to your legs. Imagine your legs relaxing more, letting go from the hips, as if the joints were getting softer. Imagine your hips relaxing.*
- *Imagine your knees relaxing. Picture that for a moment. Take a slow, full breath and relax the breath out.*
- *Check through from head to toes. Could any parts do with some more melting? Could they relax more? Stay like this for a little while.*
- *Take a slow full breath, and feel what it is like inside you now.*
  (Pause)
- *What colours would go with how you feel now?*
- *Now slowly move your toes a little and stretch your fingers. Open your eyes.*
- *Turn onto your side, curl up for a moment. Take your time. Then gently sit up.*
- Client is invited to create a mandala, showing how they feel after the activity.
- Discussion:
  - *Could you talk about how you felt before and after the relaxation?*
  - *Was it easy or difficult to concentrate on the exercise?*
  - *Which parts of your body were most relaxed?*
  - *Were there any parts that did not relax?*
  - *What are the times in your life when it would be helpful to relax?*

References

Arslan, G. (2016). Psychological maltreatment, emotional and behavioral problems in adolescents: The mediating role of resilience and self-esteem. *Child Abuse & Neglect, 52*, 200–209.

Boynton, H. M. (2016). *Navigating in seclusion: The complicated terrain of children's spirituality in trauma, grief and loss.* University of Calgary (Canada). ProQuest Dissertations & Theses, 10296321.

Boynton, H. M., & Mellan, C. (2021). Co-creating authentic sacred therapeutic space: A spiritually sensitive framework for counselling children. *Religions, 12*(7), 524.

Butler, R. J., & Gasson, S. L. (2005). Self esteem/self concept scales for children and adolescents: A review. *Child and Adolescent Mental Health Volume, 10*(4), 190–201.

Cervantes, J. M., & Arczynski, A. V. (2015). Children's spirituality: Conceptual understanding of developmental transformation. *Spirituality in Clinical Practice, 2*(4), 245–255.

Coholic, D. (2010). *Arts activities for children and young people in need: Helping children to develop mindfulness, spiritual awareness and self-esteem.* Jessica Kingsley Publishers.

Dragan, D., McDuffie, D., & Crowther, M. R. (2025). Health benefits of spirituality. In J. Uribarri & J. A. Vassalotti (Eds.), *Nutrition, fitness and mindfulness: An evidence-based guide for clinicians* (pp. 255–265). Springer Nature.

Davidson, R. J., Kabat-Zinn, J., Schumacher, J., Rosenkranz, M., Muller, D., Santorelli, S. F., Urbanowski, F., Harrington, A., Bonus, K., & Sheridan, J. F. (2003). Alterations in brain and immune function produced by mindfulness meditation. *Psychosomatic Medicine, 65*(4), 564–570.

Doyle, C., (2006) *Working with abused children: From theory to practice.* Palgrave Macmillan.

Earvolino-Ramirez, M. (2007). Resilience: A concept analysis. *Nursing Forum, 42*(2), 73–82.

Emler, N. (2001). *Self esteem: The costs and causes of low self worth.* York Publishing Services.

Erikson, E. H. (1968). *Identity: Youth and crisis* (Vol. 68). Norton.

Fosha, D. (2003). Dyadic regulation and experiential work with emotion and relatedness in trauma and disordered attachment. In D. J. Siegel & M. F. Solomon (Eds.), *Healing trauma: Attachment, trauma, the brain and the mind* (pp. 221–281). Norton.

Fredrickson, B. L., Tugade, M. M., Waugh, C. E., & Larkin, G. R. (2003). What good are positive emotions in crisis? A prospective study of resilience and emotions following the terrorist attacks on the United States on September 11th, 2001. *Journal of Personality and Social Psychology, 84*(2), 365–376.

Germer, C. K. (2005). What is it? What Does it Matter. In C. K. Germer, R. D. Siegel, & P. R. Fulton (Eds.), *Mindfulness and psychotherapy* (pp. 3–27). Guilford.

Graber, R., Pichon, F., & Carabine, E. (2015). *Psychological resilience.* Overseas Development Institute.

Greenberg, L. S. (2002). Integrating an emotion-focused approach to treatment into psychotherapy integration. *Journal of Psychotherapy Integration, 12*(2), 154–189.

Grepmair, L., Mitterlehner, F., Loew, T., & Nickel, M. (2007). Promotion of mindfulness in psychotherapists in training: Preliminary study. *European Psychiatry, 22*(8), 485–489.

Haug, I. E. (1998). Including a spiritual dimension in family therapy: Ethical considerations. *Contemporary Family Therapy, 20*, 181–194.
Heer, K. (1998). *Creative transformations: Art therapy used to develop self-esteem and spirituality in children* -(ProQuest dissertations & theses). Ursuline College..
Jacobson, J. L. (2002). *An exploratory study regarding the effects of praying for others on physical and mental health in older adults* (Doctoral dissertation). Spalding University.
Jiaa, H., & Lubetkinb, E. I. (2020). Impact of adverse childhood experiences on quality-adjusted life expectancy in the U.S. population. *Child Abuse & Neglect, 102*, 104418.
Joslin, S. J., & Gingrich, H. D. (2022). Spiritually competent counseling practice with children. *Journal of Spirituality in Mental Health, 24*(4), 381–399.
Kabat-Zinn, J. (1994). *Wherever you go, there you are: Mindfulness meditation in everyday life*. Hyperion.
King, G. A. (2004). The meaning of life experiences: Application of a meta-model to rehabilitation sciences and services. *American Journal of Orthopsychiatry, 74*(1), 72–88.
Lightsey Jr, O. R. (2006). Resilience, meaning, and well-being. *The Counseling Psychologist, 34*(1), 96–107.
Luthar, S. S., Cicchetti, D., & Becker, B. (2000). The construct of resilience: A critical evaluation and guidelines for future work. *Child Development, 71*(3), 543–562.
Maslow, A. H. (1943). A theory of human motivation. *Psychological Review, 50*, 370–396.
Masten, A. S. (2001). Ordinary magic: Resilience processes in development. *American Psychologist, 56*(3), 227–238.
McMahon, B. J. (2007). Resilience factors and processes: No longer at risk. *Alberta Journal of Educational Research, 53*(2), 127–142.
Merrick, M. T., Ports, K. A., Ford, D. C., Afifi, T. O., Gershoff, E. T., & Grogan-Kaylor, A. (2017). Unpacking the impact of adverse childhood experiences on adult mental health. *Child Abuse & Neglect, 69*, 10–19.
Paintner, C. V. (2007). The relationship between spirituality and artistic expression: Cultivating the capacity for imagining. *Spirituality in Higher Education Newsletter, 3*(2), 1–6.
Pandya, S. P. (2024). Spirituality and creativity in the early childhood context. *International Journal of Children's Spirituality, 29*(1), 18–41.
Park, E. A. (2013). *Utilizing creative and expressive therapies to explore spiritual themes with traumatized children: A family psychology perspective and theoretical formulation* (ProQuest dissertations & theses). Azusa Pacific University.
Pinquart, M., & Gerke, D-C. (2019). Associations of parenting styles with self-esteem in children and adolescents: A meta-analysis. *Journal of Child and Family Studies, 28*, 2017–2035.
Raftopoulos, M., & Bates, G. (2011). 'It's that knowing that you are not alone': The role of spirituality in adolescent resilience. *International Journal of Children's Spirituality, 16*(2), 151–167.
Rak, C. F., & Patterson, L. E. (1996). Promoting resilience in at-risk children. *Journal of Counseling & Development, 74*(4), 368–373.
Rogers, C. R. (1951). *Client-centered therapy. Its current practice, implications and theory*. Constable.
Rosenberg, M. (1965). *Society and the adolescent self-image*. Princeton University Press.

Shaffer, D. R., & Kipp, K. (2010). *Developmental psychology: Childhood and adolescence* (8th ed.). Wadsworth, Cengage Learning.
Siegel, D. (2007). *The mindful brain: Reflection and attunement in the cultivation of well-being*. W. W. Norton and Co.
Sifers, S. K., Warren, J. S., & Jackson, Y. (2012). Measuring spirituality in children. *Journal of Psychology and Christianity*, *31*(3), 209–218.
Stoltenborgh, M., Bakermans-Kranenburg, M. J., Alink, L. R., & IJzendoorn, M. H. (2012). The universality of childhood emotional abuse: A meta-analysis of worldwide prevalence. *Journal of Aggression, Maltreatment & Trauma*, *21*(8), 870–890.
Stoltenborgh, M., Bakermans-Kranenburg, M. J., Lenneke, A. & van IJzendoorn, M. H. (2014). Thep of child maltreatment across the globe: Review of a series of meta-analyses. *Child Abuse Review*, *24*(1), 37–50.
Vitorino, L. M., Lucchetti, G., Leão, F. C., Vallada, H., & Peres, M. F. P. (2018). The association between spirituality and religiousness and mental health. *Scientific Reports*, *8*(1), 17233.
Weinfield, N. S., Sroufe, L. A., Egeland, B., & Carlson, E. A. (1999). The nature of individual differences in infant–caregiver attachment. In J. Cassidy & P. R. Shaver (Eds.), *Handbook of attachment: Theory, research, and clinical applications* (pp. 68–88). The Guilford Press.
Worthington Jr, E. L., Hook, J. N., Davis, D. E., & McDaniel, M. A. (2011). Religion and spirituality. *Journal of Clinical Psychology*, *67*(2), 204–214.

Appendix A

Setting Up an Expressive Therapies Room

Checklist for an Ideal Counselling Room

Results from: Pearson, M., & Wilson, H. (2012). Soothing spaces and healing places: Is there an ideal counselling room design? *Psychotherapy in Australia*, 18(3), 46–53.

- **Choice in Seating**: e.g., lounge, chair, cushions
- **Size of the Room**: larger preferred, physical space connected to psychological space
- **Use of Colour**: creation of a calming atmosphere, emotional warmth and comfort
- **Lighting**: softer, natural light was favoured and a view of the outside
- **Privacy**: with access to the outside – ideally a natural or garden space
- **Soundproofing**: quiet with audio privacy
- **Floor Coverings**: soft
- **Fresh Air**: rather than air-conditioning (depends on humidity and comfort levels)
- **Decoration**: warm, inviting, peaceful, friendly, welcoming, uncluttered. Not too formal, not like "an office".

Some Basic Equipment

- Large cushions and/or bean bags, yoga mat
- A range of coloured pencils, pens and crayons
- Paper – A3 size
- Large clipboards for A3 paper
- Large plastic plate – for drawing mandala circles (see page 72)
- Collection of interesting stones and a candle (see page 53)
- Equipment to play or stream recorded music
- Collection of recorded music
- Music/noise-making instruments – e.g., drums (see page 122)
- Copies of the Feeling Words Lists – see below
- Textures box
- Miniatures for Symbol Work
- A3 size worksheets
- Sentence starter worksheets

Appendix B

Feeling Word Lists

These lists were created to help clients find the words that best match their feelings. When they are completing one of the exercises that asks them to think of words to go with feelings, they can scan through these lists and find the words that come closest to matching their responses.

Feeling good	*Feeling not so good*	*Feeling bad*
accepted	agitated	afraid
brave	alarmed	angry
confident	bored	annoyed
content	cautious	anxious
competent	confused	belittled
co-operative	defensive	depressed
delighted	disappointed	distrusting
elated	disillusioned	frightened
energetic	doubtful	frustrated
enthusiastic	heavy	hopeless
excited	hurt	miserable
fulfilled	hyper	nasty
genuine	ignored	psycho
happy	insecure	rejected
hopeful	inferior	sad
honest	intolerant	sorrow
impressed	jealous	spiteful
knowledgeable	jumpy	vengeful
loving	lonely	worthless
mischievous	moody	
optimistic	naughty	
overjoyed	numbed	
peaceful	overlooked	
pleased	picked on	
relaxed	resentful	
relieved	repulsed	
respectful	shame	
satisfied	shocked	

Feeling good	*Feeling not so good*	*Feeling bad*
strong	superior	
successful	suspicious	
tolerant	tense	
tough	unhappy	
trusting	unloved	
useful	wired	
valued	worried	
warmth	yearning	

Can you think of any more?

Appendix C

Shapes Page

The shapes on the following page are designed to help students think about other ways to describe feelings. When an exercise asks them to think about shapes that go with feelings, they can look over this page and choose one or two shapes, or make up their own.

Index

For Product Safety Concerns and Information please contact our
EU representative GPSR@taylorandfrancis.com Taylor & Francis
Verlag GmbH, Kaufingerstraße 24, 80331 München, Germany